OBESITY IN AYURVEDA

(A Handbook on Sthaulya Chikitsa in Ayurveda)

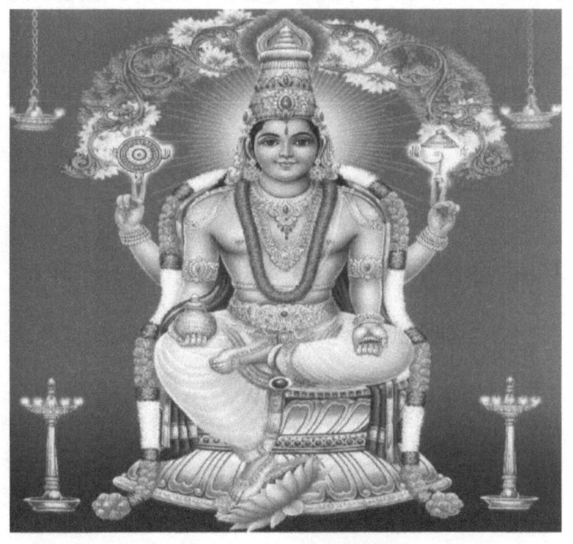

ॐ नमो भगवते महासुदर्शनाय वासुदेवाय धन्वंतरायेः
अमृतकलश हस्ताय सर्व भयविनाशाय सर्व रोगनिवारणाय
त्रिलोकपथाय त्रिलोकनाथाय श्री महाविष्णुस्वरूप
श्री धनवंतरी स्वरूप श्री श्री श्री औषधचक्र नारायणाय नमः॥

Prof. Dr. Amarprakash Dwivedi
M. S., Ph.D. (Ayu.)

RIGI PUBLICATION

All right reserved

OBESITY IN AYURVEDA

By

Prof. Dr. Amarprakash Dwivedi

Copyright© Prof. Dr. Amarprakash Dwivedi 2021

Originally published in India

Edition: 1

ISBN: 978-93-91041-06-9

Printer: Manipal Printers

Published by RIGI PUBLICATION

777, Street no.9, Krishna Nagar Khanna-141401 (Punjab), India

Website: www.rigipublication.com

Email: info@rigipublication.com

Phone: +91-9357710014, +91-9465468291

PREFACE

Sthaulya- Obesity is no more a disease but has turned into a syndrome. The extent of etiological factors is increasing day by day demanding for a root level Lifestyle modification. Pathogenesis of Sthaulya is no more confined to Rasa, Meda Dhatu but all Ardra, Snigdha constituents of body are getting involved. Prevalence since childhood age group is increasing very speedily. This takes a toll on physical and psychological growth of a person. Here, puberty related affections are dangerous as hormonal imbalance caused is considerable. This puts a nidus for abnormal and/ or underdevelopment during puberty and further for infertility.

Special concern about childhood obesity and female obesity has to be there as percentage increase in evidence is considerable. Furthermore female obesity predisposes to congenital- Hyperplastic obesity that doesn't responds well to therapies.

This book reflects our views about Sthaulya. Preventive aspect for large group of people prone to obesity is main concern. That is why, my opinions about prevention and management of childhood obesity are mentioned for expert's comments of readers.

As stated earlier, prevention and management of female obesity is my topic of special interest. Female obesity is very closely related to infertility and childhood obesity. Female body goes through lot of anatomical and physiological changes throughout life. So, special treatment plans are to be advised as per age and stage of female body. Brief mention of it will be found herein.

Judicious and genuine management of Sthaulya is done with treatment triad i.e. Drugs, Diet regulation and Exercise. Scientific elaboration of these along with small tips about the same is mentioned so as to make it more applicable rather than mere theoretical.

Enlisting of herbal drugs and herbo-mineral combinations is done so as to have wide scope for selection of drugs as per constitution, Dosha vitiation and specific for the patient and condition.

This is a humble effort to compile information as well as sharing of views and eventually formulate a Sthaulya chikitsa upakrama- a holistic plan for prevention and management of Obesity.

Thank you!

Dr. Amarprakash Dwivedi

INDEX

CHAPTER 1
CONCEPT OF OBESITY (STHAULYA)

Prakrut Meda-

Meda is viscid, greasy, fatty substance like ghrita and found in internal body. Its locations are udaranta (abdominal wall-omentum) tvachamadhya (under skin). 'Meda' is considered to be fat in general, whereas 'vasa' indicates to muscles fat. Kalas are seven in all and they are situated at the extreme borders (forming encasement and support) of the different fundamental principles of the organism.

The third kala is called medodhara. Meda is (chiefly) present in abdomen of all the animals, as well as in cartilages (small bones). The fatty substance present in large bones is as majja (marrow); whereas a substance similar in appearance and found inside other bony structures (cartilages) should be considered as meda, mixed with blood.

The persons endowed with essence of medas have particulars unctuousness (visesasneho) in complexion (varna), voice (svara), eyes (netra), hair (kesa), skin hair (loma), nail (nakha), teeth (danta), lips (oustha), urine (mutra) and faeces (purisa). This type of personality – physical profile –indicates wealth (vita), power(aisvarya), happiness (sukha), enjoyment (upabhoga), charity (dana), simplicity (arjavam) and delicacy (sukumara) in dealings (upacaratam cacaste).

Samhat Sharir-

Samhanana, samhati and samyojana are synonymous terms applied to compactness of body. A well compact body is known by smasubibhaktasthi, subaddha-sandhi. Those having well-compact body (samhata sharir) are strong.

Various standards and norms of ideal physique possessing a balanced proportion of different dhatus including meda have been set in ancient medical system as evidence by textual references referred from Charaka Samhita.

Censurable Persons - Nindita Purusah

As propounded by Lord Atreya, Agnivesa, the leading sage of Punarvasu Atreya's, discussed topic of despicable persons (nindita purusah) by covering eight types of undesirable or censurable persons (asttounindita):

Eight kinds of persons are considered to be despicable or unappreciable for their body or physical figure, such as:

    i.   Over-tall (atidirgha) ;
    ii.   Over-short (atihrsva);
    iii.   Over-hairy (atilom);
    iv.   Hairless (aloma);
    v.   Over –black (atikrishna);
    vi.   Over-fair (atigoura)
    vii. Over-obese (atisthula)
   viii. Over-lean (atikrisha)

There are two major kinds of disease viz. physical (sharira) and mental (manasa) and in present context, the normality and abnormality of physique (deha) has specially been taken into consideration.

Primarily, there are two principal locations or sites of diseases in accordance to the fundamentals of medical system:

Both body (shariram) and mind (satvam) are the locations of diseases or disorders (vyadhi) as well as pleasures (sukhanim). The balanced use or application (yoga) of time (kala), intelligence (buddhi) and sense objects (indriyartha) is cause of pleasure (sukha) which basically provides, maintains and bestows good health and pleasureful life.

But, in case of abnormalcy in body the imbalance of trio-factors has its initial role as causative factors:

Perverted, negative and excessive use of time, intelligence and sense objects is the three-fold cause (trividho hetu sangrah) of both psychic and somatic disorders (dvayashrayanam vyadhinam).

There is wide concept of classification of diseases (roga vargikarnam)

Thus, innate diseases afflict their site i.e. physique or body of person (deha) and eight types of physical discrepancies which may later lead to various kinds of diseases do occur in body. These despicable characteristics are as follow.

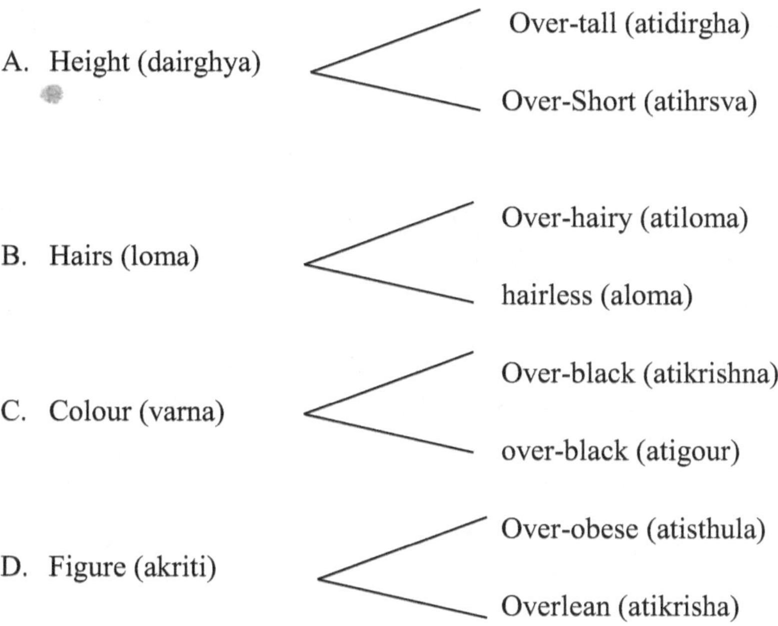

Morbidity of Meda : Prameha and Srotodusti

Death, in the form of prameha, takes away immediately the person who is dull in activites, over-obese , over-uncted and voracious eater

The person who takes food which maintains the equilibrium of dhatus (dhatusamyakarm) and also practices various physical activites, enjoys happy life.

Medovaha srotas is afflicted due to lack of physical exercise (avyayama), day-sleep (divasvapna), excessive intake of fatty food (medyana cati bhaksanat) and alocoholic driks.

Obesity-Santarpanottha Vyadhi
Sharngadhara Samhita, Purva 7, 65
Charaka Samhita, sutra 23, 3-5

One who saturates himself excessively with unctuous (snigdha), sweet (madhura), heavy (guru), slimy substances (snigdha-picchila), new cereals (navanna), fresh wine (navamada), meat of marshy and aquatic animals (mamsaiscanupavarijajaih), milk (gorasa) and its products, jiggery (guda) and flour preparations (navanna) and at the including day-sleep (divasvapna), confortable beds and seats (saiyyasana sukheratah) suffers from diseases caused by over-saturation (santrpanimittijah).

If this condition is not counteracted (sighrama pratikurvatah) promptly, (various diseases are produced such as-prameha, pidaka, jvara, kustha, amapradosa, mutrakrcchra, arochaka, tandra, klaibya, atisthoulya, alasya, gurugatrata, indriya srotasam lepa, buddhermohah, pramilaka, shopha and vividhashchanye.

Thus, the major condition of over-saturation (santarpana) is liable to cause gradually manifestation affecting functioning of various systems and this kind of pathogenesis fastly leads to produce obesity and a number of ailments depending on different factors of individuals.

In Ayurveda, Sthoulya (Obesity) is regarded as Medoroga —A disorder of Meda Dhatu- adipose tissue and fat metabolism that is one of the undesirable Constitution.

Ati Sthula has been defined as a person, "who on account of the inordinate increase of fat, is disfigured with pendulous, buttocks, belly and breasts and whose increased bulk is not matched by a corresponding increase in energy

Obesity is a medical condition in which excess body fat has accumulated to the extent that it may have an adverse effect on health, leading to reduced life expectancy and/or increased health problems

Ayurveda has proved it that it is the genomic variation that regulates the range of body weight at which set point is set. This is concept of

Prakruti. Prakruti alongwith Agni and condition of body channels i.e. srotas are responsible for setting weight at certain range. Changes in food, lifestyle and psychological changes for short duration and on a smaller scale will not affect body weight on a wider range. But, if drastic changes in Charya are there continuously for length of time, then homeostasis is lost and gaining of weight or weight loss starts. Weight gain initially leads to condition of overweight and further to obesity.

Non-practice of physical exercise or absence of physical exercise, day-sleep and intake of food increasing Shleshma, Swed (Sweat) and Snigdha (unctuousness), which resulting cause and produce fat in excess.

Consequently, meda obstructs channels causing Srotoavarodha and other body tissues-deha Dhatus do not get nourishment or remain neglected for enhancement or growth and ultimately, Meda only continues to develop constantly resulting in growth of Meda in excessive amount, extra ordinarily.

As the result (excessive growth, production and higher amount of meda-fat-excessiveness), one finds himself incapable for physical activities and body movements, becomes, thus, totally unable in any action on account of extra deposit of fat.

Vitality (alpaprano) as well as virility (punsa alpamaithunah) are also decreased, leading to gradual loss of vital power of life and sexual capability of copulation.

Meda (fat) is generally deposited in abdomen and small bones (udaresvasthisu sthitam), and hence the abdomen is increased and develops in size and shape mostly in over-obese persons.

Over-obese persons generally feel hunger in excess as extraordinary or abnormal state of hunger is one the major characteristics in obesity. There is occlusion of vayu by meda (medasavrttamargatvad) and it moves in koshtha specially, and while moving; there it stimulates gastric fire-appetite and makes absorption of ingested food faster. Then (in this way), the speedy digestion of food resolutely takes place in intestines, and it further promotes hunger consequently-person feels hunger within no time and so desires to consume more food stuffS due to abnormal appetite.

Before understanding obesity; which is pathology related with fat, let us understand physiology and metabolism of fat cells in brief.
Fat Cell Development has two things.

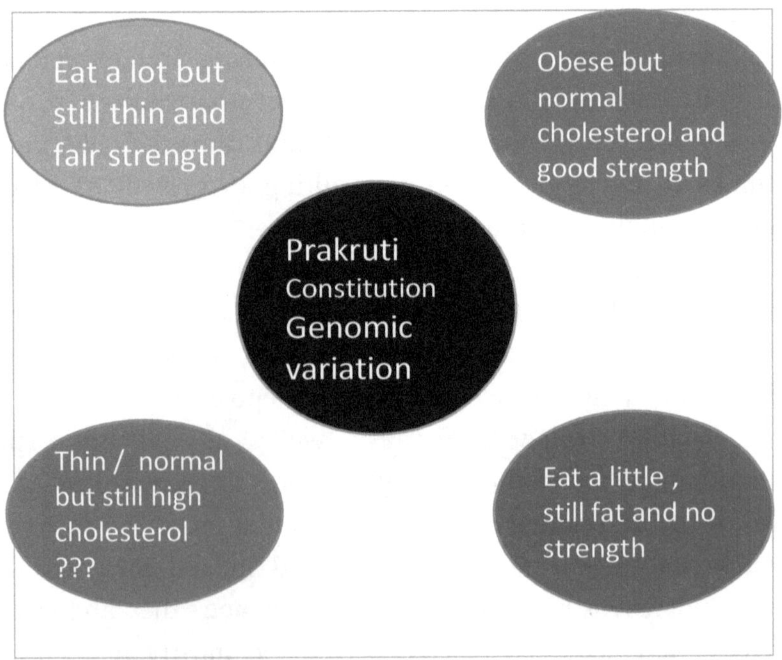

Quantitative - Increase in no. of fat cells and
Qualitative - Increase in size of fat cells.

Quantitative- Fat cell numbers increase most rapidly in later childhood and early puberty. Fat cell numbers increase in times of positive energy balance. This is called as **Hyperplastic obesity.**

Qualitative - Fat cell sizes increase when energy intake exceeds expenditure. This occurs in teenage and adulthood. This is known as **Hypertrophic obesity**

Fluctuations in weight occurs at wider range in case of Hypertrophic obesity and so, is easier to treat also. But, hyperplastic obesity is very difficult to manage and results with therapies are comparatively less.

The adverse effects of fat in non-adipose tissue are called lipotoxicity.

Fat Cell Metabolism is governed by **Lipoprotein lipase** that promotes fat storage. Men are at increased risk for developing central obesity and women are at increased risk for lower body fat.

Places in our body where fat gets accumulated are as –

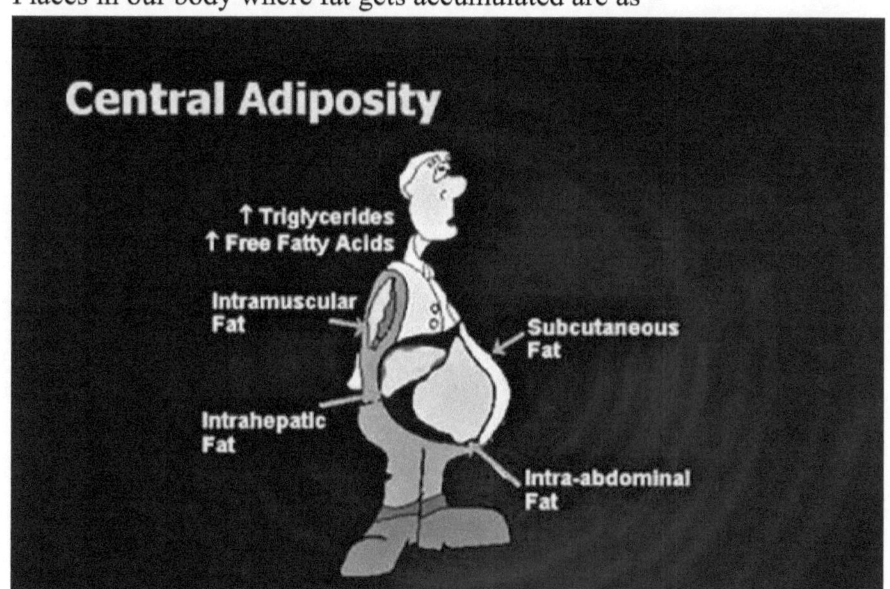

"Obesity" specifically refers to an excessive amount of **body fat**. [obesity (BMI $\geq$ 30)]Whereas, "Overweight" refers to an excessive amount of **body weight** that includes muscle, bone, fat, and water. Overweight (BMI 25-29.9)

Overweight and obesity are widespread health problems that are continuing to increase as an epidemic.

Maintenance of homeostasis – (Set-Point Theory)

Modern science believes that body has its own regulatory mechanism wherein it tries to maintain body weight at specific range. The body's natural regulatory centers maintain homeostasis at set point. If energy consumption exceeds energy expenditure, then energy storage sets in. this is mainly in form of fat that leads to obesity.

CHAPTER 2

ETIOLOGY OF OBESITY

Etiology

Bhavaprakasha, madhyakhanda,

Chikitsa prakarana 8, sthoulyadhikara 39, 1

Fat increasement or deposition of fat is caused by various major reasons viz.

i) Avyayam- Abandoning physical exercise or exertion and non-practice of physical exercise or labour-physical immobility and luxurious living without or less physical movements and activities

ii)Divaswapna- Sleeping in day

iii) Shleshmaharasevinaha- Consumption of foods enhancing phlegm

iv) Madhuro annarasah - Consuming food articles of sweet taste in excess

v) Amarasa and

vi) Prayah snehat- Excess intake of fat contained or fatty food articles and oils, ghee ,oily substances.

Thus, there are various other causative factors relating food or dietetics (ahara) and conducts (vihara) which may be considered in context of medovriddhi in accordance to ancient concept in medical system. They are indicated as

1. Atisampuranad - Excessive intake of food (ingestion or consuming diet in abnormally higher quantity more than normal quantity of dietetic food material

2. Guru Madhura, Shita, Snigdhopayogad- Use of heavy, sweet, cold and unctuous food articles in diet in excess quantity as regular practice-with predominance or preference to fatty substances in food

3. Divasvapna- Habitual act of sleeping in day comfortably-rather for long period . Day sleep is unctuous (snigdha). By day-sleep

in seasons other than summer, kapha and pitta are vitiated, hence day-sleep is not indicated in those seasons.

4. Avyayamad- Avoidance of physical exercise and exertion of physique.
5. Avyavayad- Abstinence from performance of sex. Regularly avoiding physical activities as exerted in sexual behavior
6. Harshanityatvad- Psychological state with pleasure and happiness by all means, maximum feeling of exhilaration leading joyful life keeping always quite happy.
7. Achintanad- No worry, tension, stress and anxiety. Leading life without any kind of mental fatigue, pressure or burden of psychological adverse feeling e.g. agony, problematic matters involving mental thinking constantly lack of mental work
8. Beejasvabhavat- Genetic defect inherited from the parents i.e. either father or mother and both affecting their child.

    In this manner excessive increase of fat results due to meda vardhaka and kaphavardhaka aahara and vihara when they are taken or followed.

Causes of Sthaulya are divided as-
1. Dietary causes- Aharaj Hetu
2. Lifestyle related causes- Viharaj Hetu
3. Genetical – Beejswabhavat
4. disease and drugs related- Aagantuj Hetu
5. Psychological factors- Manasik Hetu
6. Miscellaneous - Anya

Aharaja Hetu-
Gunapradhana - Guru, Sheeta, Pichchila, Snigdha.
Rasapradhana - Madhura.
Dravyapradhana - Navanna, Gorasa, Dadhi, Atimeda, Goudika, Varuni, Anupavarija mamsa.
Vidhipradhana- Adhyasana, Atisampoorna, Atimatra ahara.
Dietary causes-
Present and past eating; influences current body weight.

Dietary causes are mainly of 2 types-

1] Overeating

2] Changes in food habbits

- Increased energy intake – increased Portion sizes. Serving a larger portion of a beverages increases beverage consumption
- Snacking with loss of regular meals
- Energy – dense food (mainly fat)
- Since the 1960s the industry has increased the single-serving size from a standard 6-½-ounce bottle to a 20- ounce bottle.
- With increased calorie-containing beverages, energy intake increases
- increased media advertising
- Increased availability of energy-dense foods
- Increased cost of fruits and vegetables
- Increased caloric intake when eating out
- Increased consumption of soft drinks
- Reduced consumption of fruits and vegetables
- Reduced frequency of family meals
- Restrained eating, meal skipping
- Over eating
- Frequent food intake before digestion of a previous meal.
- Kapha increasing food
- Excessive consumption of sweet food, Heavy food, cold diet, unctuous food –like dairy products- cheese cream butter, ice cream yogurt
- Excess use of oily food-fried food grilled food, fast foods
- Excessive use of meat
- SSB Consumption Trends
- Usage of new grains
- Usage of preparations of sugarcane, jaggery.
- Excessive use of Rice, wheat, Black gram,
- Drinking water after food in take
- Cultural Factors –Type of food ,way of cooking is different.

- Increased availability of convenient food, large portions, and energy-dense foods
- (before party, tell body that you will be eating more, so it responses by increasing metabolic rate, secretion of digestive juices, enzymes & blood flow to your stomach.)

Viharaja Hetu-

Avyayma, Shayyasana sukha, Diwaswapna, Cheshta dwesha.

- Decreasing energy expenditure
- insufficient sleep, insomnia
- **Life style and behavior**
- Sedentary life style – physical inactivity
- Lack of physical exercise
- excessive sleep mainly at day time and soon after meal
- Lack of sexual life,
- Modern technology replaces physical activities.
- Physical activity is important to allow people to eat enough food to get needed nutrients.

Manasika Hetu-

Achinta, Arati, Harshanityatwa.

- Lack of thinking,
- anxiety or anger.
- Cheerful mind
- finding no means of self expression
- depression

STRESS

- **Stress** leads to secretion of cortisol in our body that lowers metabolic rate, prevents fat burning & help convert food to fat. We can reduce cortisol production by leading disciplined lives. (Achar Rasayan)

Beejaswabhavat (Genetic Factors) -

- **Genetics -** Leptin (also called the ob protein)

- Protein Produced by fat cells under the direction of the ob gene that acts as a hormone to increase energy expenditure and decrease appetite and May be deficient in obese individuals
- **Environment- Race**– The gene pool of our population remains relatively unchanged.
- **'Beeja Svabhavat'** Irrespective of diet the person is obese due to genetic makeup.
- Natural selection for higher BMI.
- Epigenetic risk factors passed on generationally,

Aagantuja Hetu- Disease and drug related -

Related with disease-

- Diseases like Hypothyroidism,
- Cushing syndrome,
- Polycystic ovarian syndrome
- Hypothalamic tumours-
- insulinoma.

Related with drugs-

- Drug – Tricyclic antidepressants, Sodium valproate
- Corticosteroids- Estrogen containing OC pills
- Sulphonylureas,
- B – Blockers.

Other (Anya) –

- Social Factors- poverty and a lower level of education
- **Pregnancy at a later age** (which may cause susceptibility to obesity in children).

Homeostasis of weight management is maintained by balance in energy consumption and energy expenditure.

CHAPTER 3

MANIFESTATIONS OF OBESITY

Symptomatology

Person possessing fat in excess begins to develop various sings and symptoms, viz.

i) Khsudra shvasa

ii) Trishna (thirst in excess)

iii) Moha

iv) Nidra

v) Krthanam-ucchvasavarodha

vi) Kanthaghurghura

vii) Glani

viii) Kshudha (appetite in excess)

ix) Dehadourgandhya (unpleasant body odour)

x) Alpaprana (lesser vitality and weak in general); and

xi) Alpamaithuna (incapability or insufficiency in performing sexual act)

xii) Udara Vriddhi (Location of meda or fat is abdomen or belly of peoples hence, belly is generally increased in over-obese persons.)

Major Defects of Over-Obese –

There are eight defects chiefly which are reflected over human body of over-obese persons, viz.

i) **Ayushohrasa** - Life span of over-obese person becomes short

ii) **Javoparodha** - Movement or activities of body in routine become hampered, with loss of enthusiastic activity of human body showing laziness in any bodily action;

iii) **Krichravyavaya** - Feeling difficulty in performance of sexual intercourse by showing physical inactivity in sexual act to full extent;

iv) **Dourbalya** - Person suffers from debility in general

v) **Dourgandhya** - Body of person given foul smell

vi) **Swedabadha** - Whole body of person is over-sweating or sweating in excess (abnormally) causes uneasiness to person

vii) **Kshudatimatra** - Person experiences excessive hunger and

viii) **Pipasaatiyoga** - Person remains over-thirsty .

Thus, major characteristics observed in the anomalistic condition of obesity are highlighted in description of ati-sthoulya (over-obese) given by Agnivesha who has paid attention mainly towards salient features of obesity in the form of defects (dosha or vikriti). These are often experienced, more or less depending upon different factors and individuals as well as extent of excess quantity of meda. Abnormalcy is mainly of two kinds, one relates to various signs and symptoms and another pertains to long term adverse effects.

STHOULYA ROOPA-
- Udara,Stana,Sphik lambana
- Udara,Stana,Sphik chalatwa
- Dourbalya
- Kshudraswasa
- Atinidra
- Krathana
- Gadgadatwa
- Ghananga
- Trishna
- Moha
- Galatalu shosha
- Anga daha , Kara pada daha
- Madhurasya
- Hritnetra jihwa shravana upalepa
- Shitilanga
- Shayyasana, swapna, sukha
- Sheetapreeti
- Keshanakha ativrudhi, Ayatha utsaha.

CHAPTER 4

TYPES OF OBESITY

Obesity is a medical condition in which excess body fat has accumulated to the extent that it may have an adverse effect on health, leading to reduced life expectancy and/or increased health problems

Obesity is divided in different types as per causative factors i. e. etiology, pathogenesis, distribution and sites of deposition of excess fat.

Types –

1.) Types on basis of aetiology-

       1. Primary / Simple / Exogenous

       2. Secondary / Endogenous.

2.)Types on basis of histopathology-

1. Hyperplastic- increase in adipocyte number. This continues lifelong and has bad prognosis as weight Loss is not achieved.

2. Hypertrophic- increase in adipocyte size. This has adult onset because of storage of additional energy. It has good prognosis as weight Loss can be achieved to a great extent with different regimes.

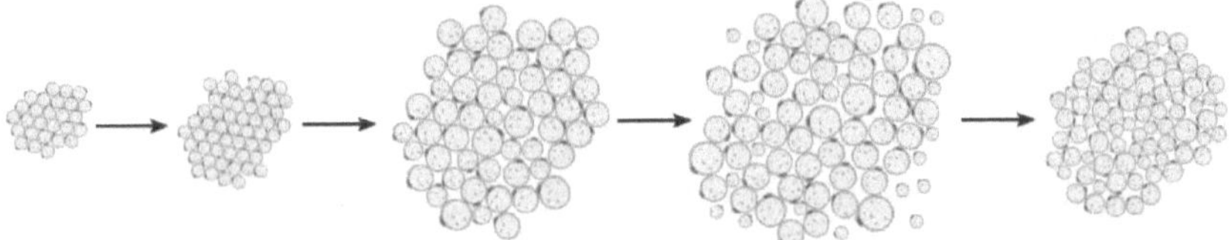

<table>
<tr><td>During growth, fat cells increase in number in later childhood, early puberty & in + energy balance

Hyper-plastic</td><td>When energy intake exceeds expenditure, fat cells increase in size.

Hypertro-phic</td><td>When fat cells have enlarged and energy intake continues to exceed energy expenditure, fat cells increase in number again. Adverse effect of fat in non adipose tissue is Lipotoxicity.</td><td>.With fat loss, the size of the fat cells shrinks but not the number.</td></tr>
</table>

3.) Types on basis of fat distribution--
1. Generalized
2. Central/ truncal-
   on trunk and neck- cushing and hypothyroid
3. Superior/ buffalo-
   face, neck, arm and upper trunk—cushing and hypothyroid
4. Inferior/ lypodystrophy-
   lower trunk and leg with wasting of upper body
5. Girdle, fatty apron-
   hips, buttocks and abdomen—pituitary, hypothalamic lesions
6. Breeches/ trochanteric—
   only buttocks- hypogonadal syndrome
7. Lipomatous/ multiple lipomatous –
   localized deposits of fat

4.) Types on basis of mode of onset & clinical appearance—
1. Primary/Childhood/Generalized
   Central/abdominal/Visceral/android apple-shaped –
   Here , deposition of fat is mainly on abdomen. Intra-abdominal fat gives apperance of apple. This type is common in men.
2. Secondary/Adult/Central
   Generalised/gynoid/pear shaped.-

In this type, subcutaneous fat accumulation is more. Mainly lower part of body has fat deposits. This type is more common in female. Deposition of fat in lower abdomen and thigh gives appearance like pear.

Consequences of excess deposits of fat are linked mainly to amount of **INTRA-ABDOMINAL FAT** rather than lower body fat or subcutaneous abdominal fat.

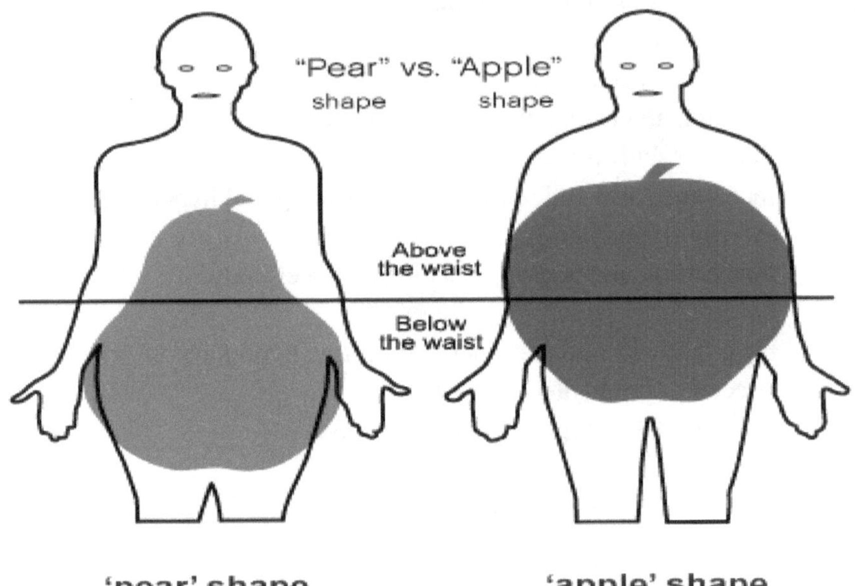

Apple-shaped people whose fat is concentrated mostly in the abdomen are more likely to develop many of the health problems associated with obesity. They are at increased health risk because of their fat distribution. While obesity of any kind is a health risk, it is better to be a pear than an apple.

PEAR - LESS DANGEROUS - DIFFICULT TO REDUCE
APPLE - DANGEROUS - EASILY REDUCIBLE

CHAPTER 5

PATHOGENESIS OF OBESITY

Consequent to various causative factors , medas is increased excessively   and meda obstructs channels or passages (meda savrittamargatvat) and further results in obstructing nourishment process of other dhatus and meda further continues to deposit in excess, which makes person quite unable in all the physical activities or body movements in general.

There is excess of fat in body and further only fat is accumulated and not the other dhatus. Thus the life is shortened. Because of laxity (shaithilya), softness and heaviness of fat; there is hampering of movement . Due to non-abundance of semen and passage having been covered with fat (avrittamargatvat), there is difficulty in sexual intercourse (Kricchravyavayata); due to disequilibrium of dhatus or connective tissues of body, there is debility. Foul smell is due to defect and nature of fat (dourgandhyam medodosham medasah svabhavat svedanattvatch) and also sweatening, due to association of medas with kapha (medasahshleshmasansargat), its oozing nature (vishyandi). Abundance (bahutva), heaviness (gurutva) and intolerance to physical execise. Because of intensified agni or indigestion (tikshnagnitvat) and abundance of vayu in belly (prabhutakoshthavayutvatccha), there is excessive hunger and thirst (kshudatimatram pipasatiyogashcheti).

In this way, the fat is deposited in excess and various characteristics in human body are produced and observed.
The person is called over-obese who due to excessive increase of fat and muscles, has pendulous buttocks, abdomen and breasts and suffers from deficient metabolism and energy. The over-obese (atisthula) and over-lean (atikrsa) are constantly indisposed and such have to be managed constantly with karshana and brinhana measures respecively.

STHAULYA SAMPRAPTI

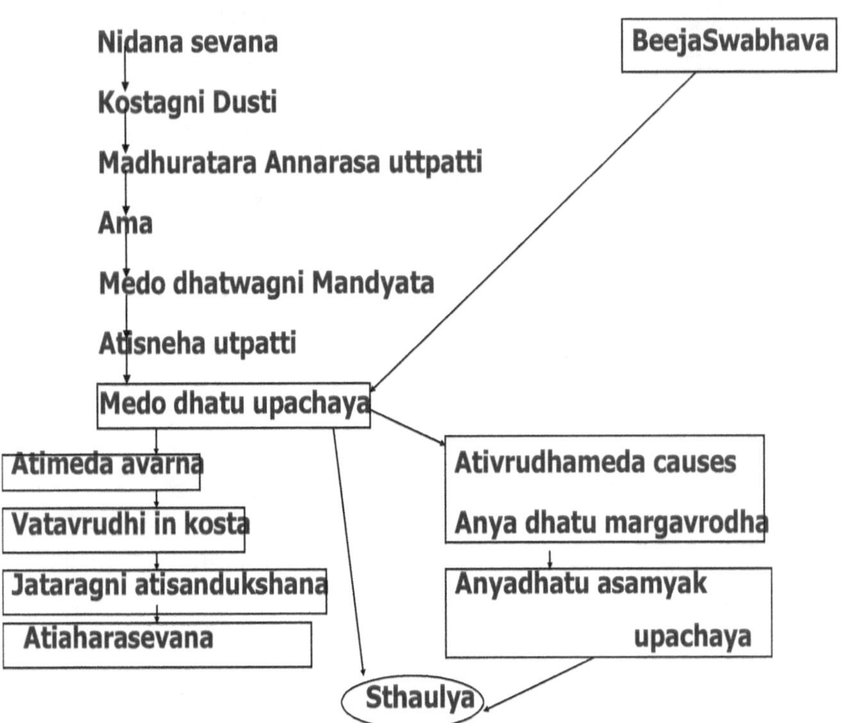

SAMPRAPTI GHATAK

Dosha	:	Kapha pradhana Vata pittanubandhi
Dooshya	:	Rasa, Mamsa, Meda
Agni	:	Jataragni, Medodhatvagni
Ama	:	Jataragnimandyajanita Ama, Medodhatvagnimandyajanita ama
Srotodusti	:	Medavaha srotas
prakara	:	Sanga
Udbhava sthana	:	Amashaya
Sanchara sthana	:	Rasayani
Adhistana	:	Medodhara kala, Vapavahana

Vyakta sthana	:	**Sarvashareera (Especially Sphik, Stana&Udara)**
Roga marga	:	**Bahya & Abhyantara**
Roga swabhava	:	**Chirakari**

Medoroga pathogenesis

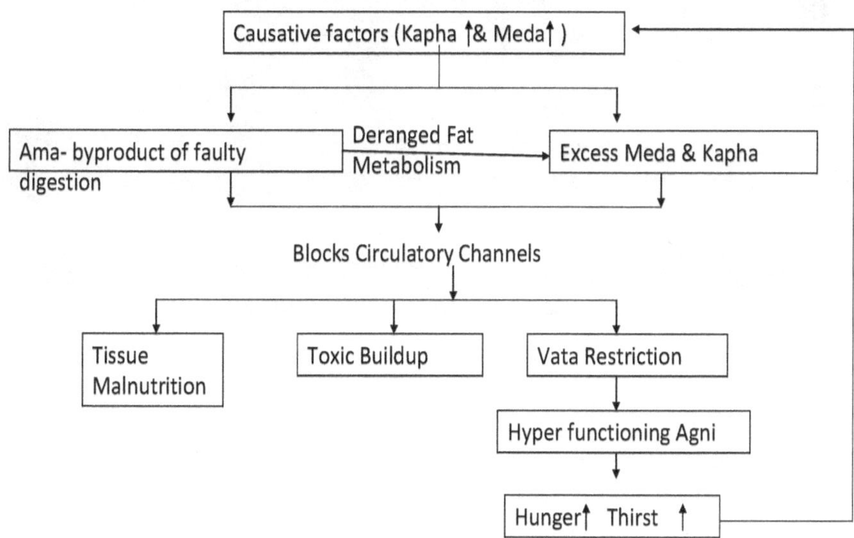

PATHOGENESIS-

Obesity especially intra-abdominal adiposity is associated with increased free fatty acid (FFA) concentration in plasma which exercises major negative effect on insulin sensitivity in both muscle and liver. Besides insulin resistance, both lipotoxicity and glucotoxicity may initiate and enable a vicious circle dependable for metabolic impairment.

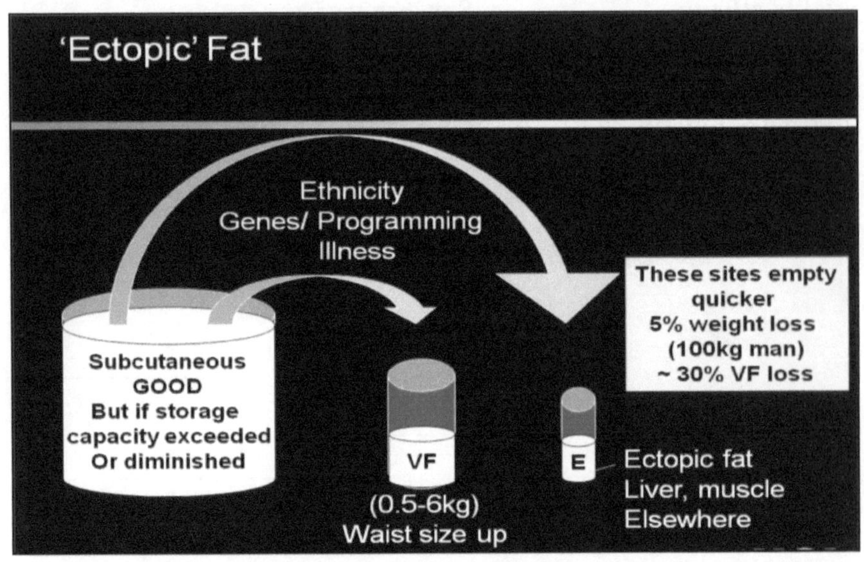
'Ectopic' Fat
Ethnicity
Genes/ Programming
Illness
Subcutaneous
GOOD
But if storage
capacity exceeded
Or diminished
These sites empty
quicker
5% weight loss
(100kg man)
~ 30% VF loss
VF
(0.5-6kg)
Waist size up
E
Ectopic fat
Liver, muscle
Elsewhere

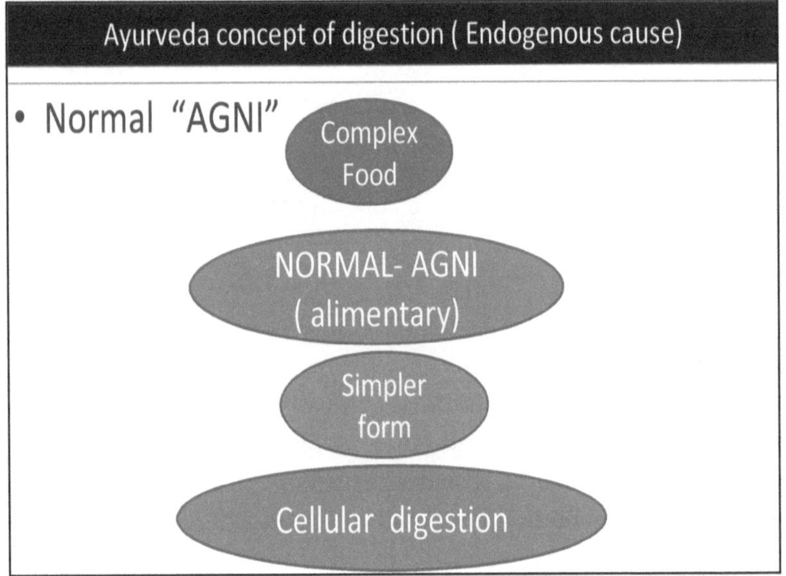
Ayurveda concept of digestion (Endogenous cause)
• Normal "AGNI"
Complex Food
NORMAL- AGNI (alimentary)
Simpler form
Cellular digestion

CONCEPT OF AGNI

TYPE OF AGNI	FOOD HABIT	BODY CONSTITUTION	STRENGTH
TEEKSHNAGNI	EAT A LOT	THIN	STRONG
(PITTA ++)		THIN	NO STRENGTH
		OVERWEIGHT	STRONG
		OVERWEIGHT	NO STRENGTH
MANDAGNI	EAT LITTLE	THIN	STRONG
(KAPHA++)		THIN	NO STRENGTH
		OVERWEIGHT	STRONG
		OVERWEIGHT	NO STRENGTH
VISHAMAGNI (VATA++)	VARIABLE QUANTITY	WEIGHT ALSO VARIATES	STRENGTH VARIATES
SAMAGNI	REGULAR MEDIUM QUANTITY	SWASTHA SHARIR	STRONG

Special points about pathogenesis--

- Indians have shorter height. Lower BMI but higher body fat content.
- Waist circumference is lower but chest and abdominal fat is higher.
- Excess fat in Indians generates more inflammatory molecules, which significantly contribute to cardiac disease.
- Genetic influence regarding obesity is there throughout life.
- In childhood, overnutrition, behavioural influences, lack of physical activity leads to obesity and starts insulin resistance.
- Obese child is likely to become obese adult. Weight tends to increase through adult life, as BMR and physical activity decreases.

CHAPTER 6
ASSESSMENT AND HAZARDS OF OBESITY

ASSESSMENT OF OBESITY

1. Body Mass index

Body Mass Index (BMI) is a number calculated from a weight and height. BMI is a reliable indicator of body fatness for most children and teens. BMI does not measure body fat directly, but correlates to direct measures of body fat, such as underwater weighing and dual energy x-ray absorptiometry (DXA).

It is calculated by dividing person's weight in kilogram by his height in meter squares

BMI	19-25	Normal range
BMI	26-30	Over Weight
BMI	30 and higher	Obese
BMI	40 and higher	Extremely Obese

Sr. No.	BMI	Prediction
1	19-25	Normal range
2	26-30	Over Weight
3	30 and higher	Obese
4	40 and higher	Extremely Obese

2. Waist to Hip ratio

- Male — Female — Health Risk
- 0.90 or below — 0.80 or below — Low Risk
- 0.96 to 1.0 — 0.81 to 0.85 — Moderate Risk
- 1.0+ — 0.85+ — High Risk

Sr. No.	Male	Female	Health Risk
1	0.90 or below	0.80 or below	Low Risk
2	0.96 to 1.0	0.81 to 0.85	Moderate Risk
3	1.0+	0.85+	High Risk

3. Waist Circumference
- Men > 40 inches
- women > 35 inches

Above these values, it is considered to have health risk.

4. Maternal weight Gain in adolescents

Distribution and percent high maternal weight gain
(>40 lb) of singleton births

Sr. No.	Maternal Age	% High maternal WG
1	<15	28.7
2	16-17	27.8
3	18-19	26.7

HAZARDS OF OBESITY

As a consequent complication of excessive increase in meda, all the three doshas e.g. vata, pitta and kapha suddenly get aggravated and it results in manifestation of a number of ailments of serious nature which may lead to condition of gravity-threat to life –for such over-obese person.

Medoroga (Obesity) Consequences

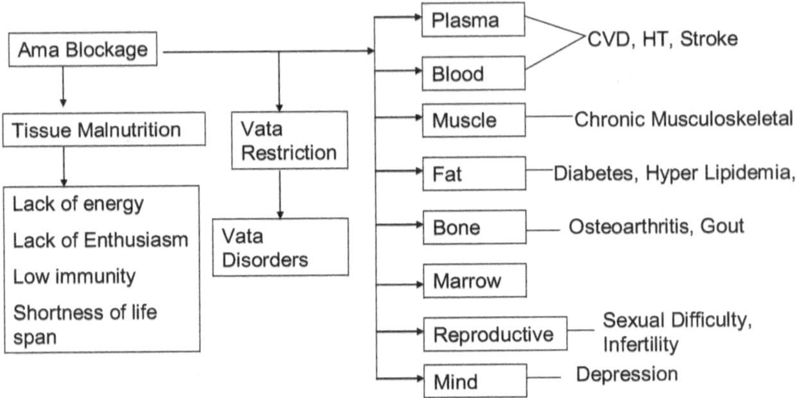

Medoroga Upadrava-
Prameha, Pidaka, Jwara, Bhagandara, Vidrudhi, Vata roga, Udara Urusthambha, Kustha, Visarpam, Atisara, Arsha, Shleepada, Apachi, Kamala, Krimi, Trusha, Moha, Vrana, Mootra krichra, Kasa, Swasa.

Prevalence, percentage and severity of obesity is increasing rapidly. Percentage of early onset of obesity is also increasing. Unfortunately , prognosis is bad in this type of Hyperplastic obesity. Furthermore, due to lifestyle changes and increasing stress, prognosis of adult onset obesity is also not very satisfactory.

This sets in a vicious cycle of obesity, obesity induced health risks, bad prognosis of obesity and side effects of treatment plans also.

- Hazards of Obesity depend on many factors such as the extent of overweight, age, health status and genetic makeup.
- Risk factors may differ among individuals.

Health risks of obesity can be differentiated and enlisted as follows-

1. **Physical**
2. **Psychological**
3. **Social**
4. **Occupational**
5. **Related with specific stages like pregnancy and post partum period.**

Extreme Obesity is Increasing Rapidly

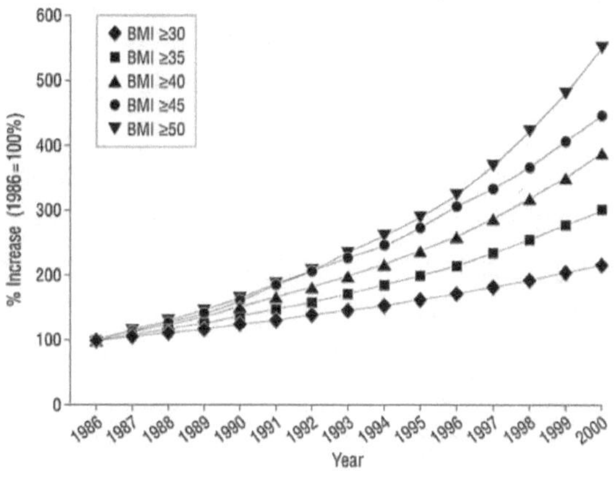

Sturm R. *Arch Intern Med* 2003;163:2146-48

1. Physical consequences as per different systems are—

A] Metabolic disorders (DM, Gall stones, Gout, Hyperlipidaemia)

B] Mechanical disabilities (OA, Hernia, Varicosity, Dysnoea, Accidents).

C] Respiratory Complications (Dysnoea, Apnoea, Pickwickian syndrome, OHS, Resp. infections).

D] Cardiovascular complications (Stroke, Venous stasis, CCF etc.).

Hazards of Obesity -

- Cardiology- Hypertension, Dyslipidaemia (abnormal cholesterol levels), ischemic heart disease, angina and myocardial infarction , congestive heart failure, , deep vein thrombosis and pulmonary embolism
- Endocrinology and – DM, Some types of cancers, thyroid dysfunction, hormonal imbalance.
- Reproductive- PCOD, menstrual disorder, infertility,complications during pregnancy, birth defects intrauterine fetal death, Post partum weight retention can lead to obesity,Hypertension,Heart disease,Diabetes,
- Dermatology- stretch marks, acanthosis nigricans, lymphedema, cellulitis, Hirsutism , intertrigo
- Gastrointestinal- GERD, fatty liver disease, cholelithiasis (gallstones), gastroesophageal reflux disease
- Neurology- Stroke, neuralgia, migraines, carpal tunnel syndrome, dementia,
  idiopathic intracranial hypertension, multiple sclerosis
- Oncology- breast, ovarian, esophageal, colorectal, liver, pancreatic, gallbladder, stomach, endometrial, cervical, prostate, kidney, non- Hodgkin's lymphoma, multiple myeloma. endometrial, cervical
- Respirology- obstructive sleep apnea, obesity hypoventilation syndrome asthma
- Increased complications during general anaesthesia
- Skeletal system- Osteoarthritis, Gout
- Pulmonary (breathing) problems, sleep apnea.
- Reproductive problems in women, including menstrual irregularities, infertility.

System	Condition	System	Condition
Cardiology	<ul><li>Hypertension,</li><li>Dyslipidaemia (abnormal cholesterol levels),</li><li>ischemic heart disease,</li><li>angina and</li><li>myocardial infarction</li><li>congestive heart failure,</li><li>deep vein thrombosis</li><li>pulmonary embolism</li></ul>	Dermatology	<ul><li>stretch marks,</li><li>acanthosis nigricans,</li><li>lymphedema,</li><li>cellulitis,</li><li>Hirsutism ,</li><li>intertrigo</li></ul>
Endocrinology and Reproductive medicine	<ul><li>Diabetes mellitus polycystic ovarian syndrome</li><li>menstrual disorder infertility</li><li>complications during pregnancy</li><li>birth defects</li><li>intrauterine fetal death</li></ul>	Gastrointestinal	<ul><li>GERD,</li><li>fatty liver disease</li><li>cholelithiasis (gallstones)</li><li>gastroesophageal reflux disease</li></ul>
Neurology	<ul><li>Stroke</li><li>Neuralgia paresthetica</li><li>Migraines</li><li>Carpal tunnel syndrome</li><li>Dementia</li><li>Idiopathic intracranial hypertension</li><li>multiple sclerosis</li></ul>	Oncology	<ul><li>breast, ovarian</li><li>esophageal, colorectal</li><li>liver, pancreatic</li><li>gallbladder, stomach</li></ul>
Psychiatry	<ul><li>depression in women</li><li>social stigmatization</li></ul>	Respirology	<ul><li>obstructive sleep apnea</li><li>obesity hypoventilation syndrome</li><li>asthma</li></ul> increased complications during general anaesthesia

1. **Psychological Problems**
- Feelings of rejection, shame and depression are common.
- Ineffective treatments can lead to a sense of failure.
- Fad Diets

- Inadequate diets
- Perceptions and Prejudices
- **Depression**
- Disappointment in love relationships
- Fear of competition
- Fear of heterosexuality
- Inability to deal with negative affect.
- Feelings of being unloved/unloveable

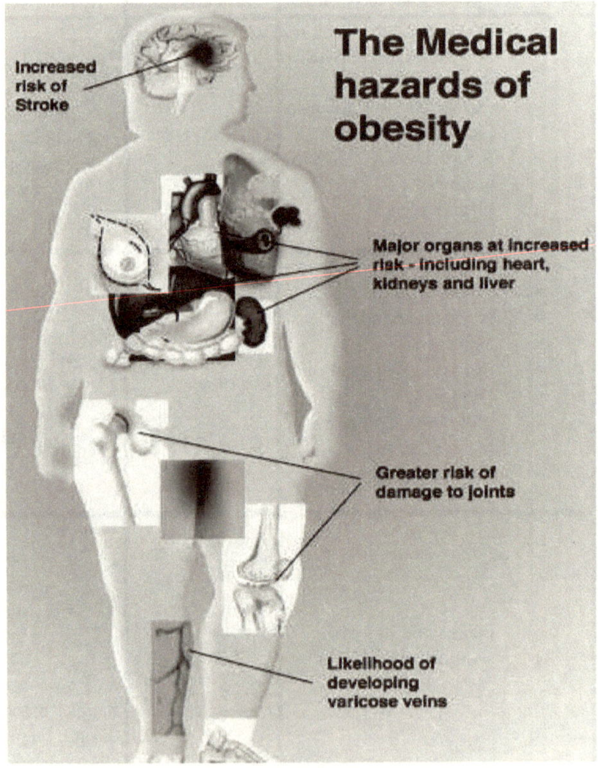

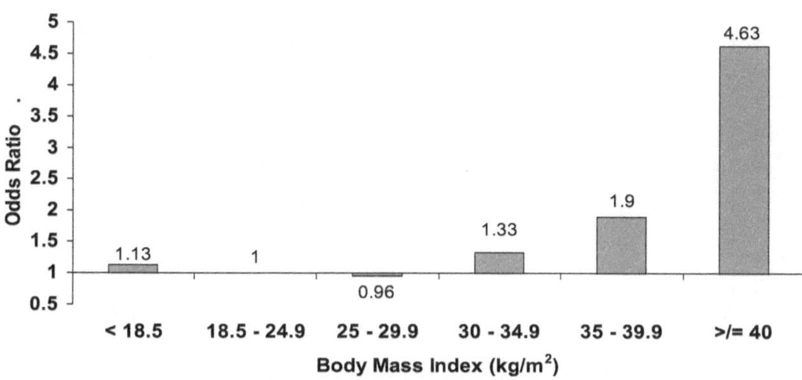

2. Social Consequences

- Prejudices and discrimination
- Judged on appearance rather than character
- Stereotyped as lazy and lacking self-control
- social stigmatization

3. Related with specific stages like pregnancy and post partum period.

- Pregnancy related health risks
- Labor and delivery complications
- Maternal anemia
- Preterm labour
- Macrosomia
- Infant Mortality

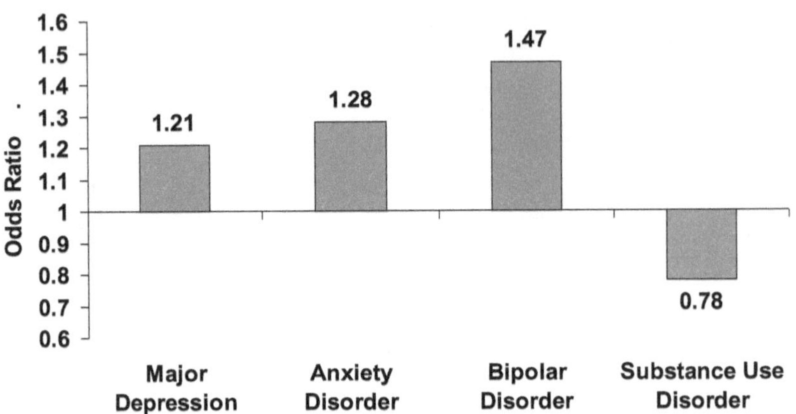

4. Post-partum weight retention and consequences

- Obesity
- Hypertension
- Heart disease
- Diabetes
- Some types of cancers

CHAPTER 7

CHILDHOOD OBESITY

Changing diet and **decreasing physical activity** are believed to be the two most important factors in causing the recent increase in the rates of obesity in children. Childhood obesity leads to insulin resistance and compensatory hyperinsulinaemia Childhood obesity often persists into adulthood and is associated with numerous chronic illnesses. So, children who are obese are often tested for hypertension, diabetes, hyperlipidemia, and fatty liver, medical complications, most worrisome metabolic risk factors.

Other main cause of childhood obesity is **Heredity & biochemical individuality– slow BMR–** lesser energy generating fat— lesser mitochondria generating energy through fat burning in metabolism.

Effects on puberty-

Puberty is a complex process by which children develop secondary sex characters and reproductive competence. It is initiated centrally, with gonadal function being driven by increased gonadotropin-releasing hormone (GnRH) and gonadotropin secretion.Adequate nutritional status is requisite for central initiation of puberty. Excess adiposity influences various aspects of pubertal development like pubertal initiation and hormonal parameters during puberty.Obesity during pubertal transition also promotes development of adolescent PCOS. As already stated physical and psychological consequences are more damaging.

Prevalence of Childhood obesity -
The percentage of overweight youth has more than doubled in the past 30
years.

- Obesity is one of the most pressing health threats to families and children nationwide.
- Large % of children and adolescents are either obese or at risk of being obese.

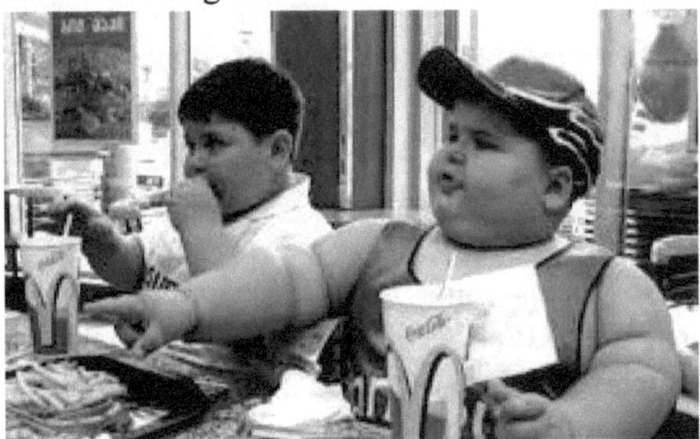

What is BMI?
Body Mass Index (BMI) is a number calculated from a child's
weight and height. BMI is a reliable indicator of body fatness for
most children and teens. BMI does not measure body fat directly, but
correlates to direct measures of body fat, such as underwater
weighing and dual energy x-ray absorptiometry (DXA).
Additionally, for children and teens, BMI is age- and sex-specific
and is often referred to as BMI-for-age.

What is BMI percentile?
After BMI is calculated for children and teens, the BMI number
is plotted on the CDC BMI-for-age growth charts (for either girls or
boys) to obtain a percentile ranking. Percentiles are the most
commonly used indicators to assess the size and growth patterns of
individual children. The percentile indicates the relative position of
the child's BMI number among children of the same sex and age.
The growth charts show the weight status categories used with

children and teens (underweight, healthy weight, at risk of overweight, and overweight).

BMI-for-age weight status categories and the corresponding percentiles are shown in the following table.

Weight Status Category	Percentile Range
Underweight	Less than the 5th percentile
Healthy weight	5th percentile to less than the 85th percentile
At risk of overweight	85th to less than the 95th percentile
Overweight	Equal to or greater than the 95th percentile

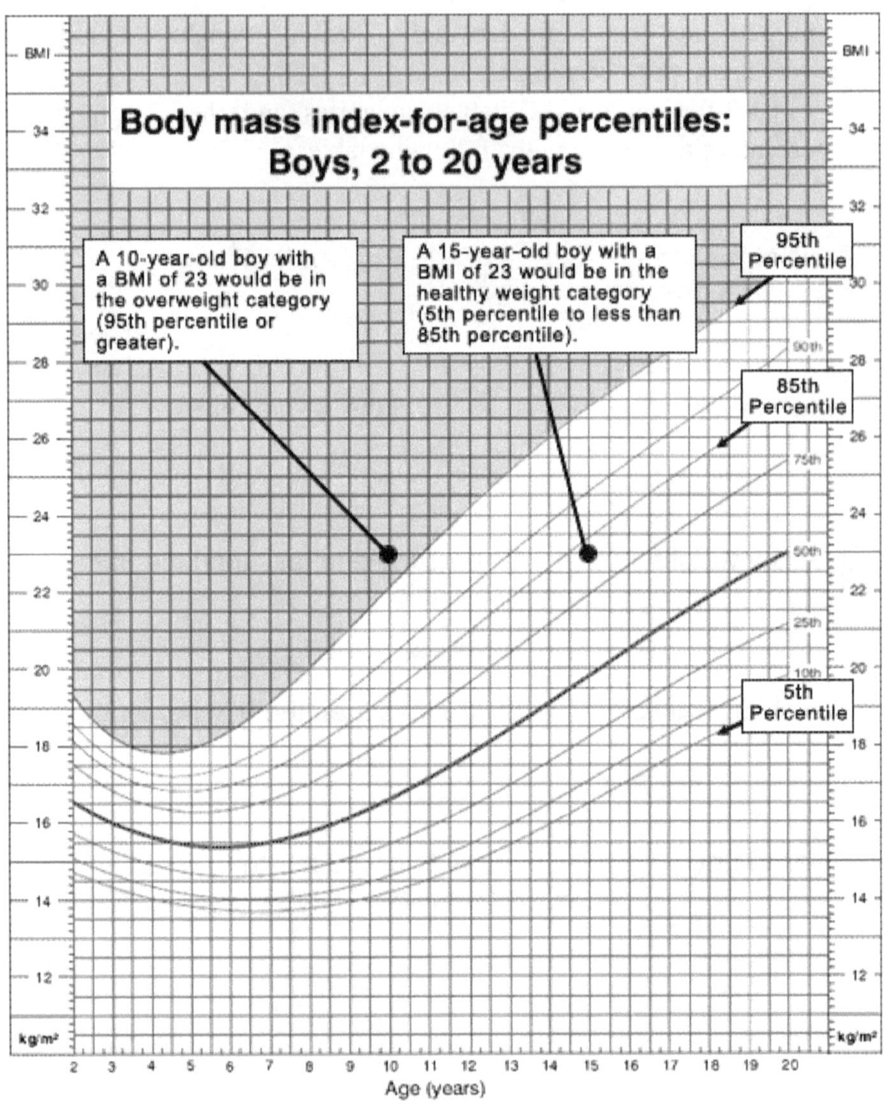

Management of Childhood Obesity-

<u>Objectives</u>--

- Become aware of childhood obesity problem
- Inform what BMI is
- At home, Consider changes that can be made

- At school level, Give ways to encourage classroom activities
- Social awareness
- Treatments used in children are primarily **lifestyle interventions and behavioral techniques.** Adopting healthy behaviors, such as following a healthy eating plan.
- Participating in regular physical activity, can help individuals achieve or maintain a healthy weight.
- Decreasing television viewing
- **Medications are not FDA approved for use in this age group.**

AT HOME-

It is very important that parents are a role model for their children.

 Behavior is learned from observation. The behaviors our kids may pick-up on, can affect their eating habits now and in the future. Therefore, we should think about our own eating regimen to support our child's positive food choices.

Ways to be a role model would be:

- Never skip meals
- Limit junk food in the house
- Eat and prepare food with children
- Try new foods but don't force children to try
- Turn off the tv while eating
- No crash diets and fear for food.
- No aerated beverages instead of water.
- Be active ourselves.

Ways to encourage better eating habits for child

- Offer kid-size servings
- Give your child a good start with breakfast
- Encourage drinking low fat milk & water
- Plan afternoon snacks
- Pay attention to hunger cues
- Avoid skipping meals

What are healthy foods

Healthy foods are those that are **nutrient-rich** or have a large amount of key vitamins and minerals for their calories. We don't have to give up our favorite foods to eat a healthy diet just try to have our core choices nutrient-rich and round out with other foods. Colorful fruits and vegetables have more nutrients, lean meats, beans, low fat and fat free dairy and nuts are examples of ideal foods.

No food is either GOOD or BAD. If we label it so, then it can restrict eating or lead to negative attitudes towards food. It is critical to make each calorie count; especially when weight may be an issue.

Prevention of CHILDHOOD OBESITY-

Concept of beejshuddhi-In some families, obesity and overweight runs as a hereditary disorder in generations together. In such cases, Prior to conception; couple can follow special charya i.e. lifestyle modifications. In addition, special panchkarma procedures should be undergone to achieve Beejshuddhi. If this is practised for at least 7 generations; Beejadoshaja sthaulya can be prevented, treated upto level of satisfaction. More or less effect will be seen in every generation.

1.For foetus (infantile origin of adult disease)-
Modified Garbhini Paricharya and GARBHASANSKAR can be advised to pregnant female to avoid excess deposition of fat especially subcutaneous fat in foetus.
2. For infants -
Use of BALRASAYAN i.e. GUTI (GHISARA)
Increase breast feeding initiation, duration, and exclusivity.

3. Toddlers, Preschoolars-
Suvarnaprashan- This special regimen will ensure healthy physical, psychological, intellectual gowth of child by dhatu poshan and balancing dhatvagni.

4. School going children-

Lifestyle designing such as to make children more active physically. This includes-

- Setting time limits on TV, video games & computers.

 encourage daily physical activity after school activities: play outdoors, walk the dog, toss a ball. provide opportunities to experience different activities & let them choose what they like. make sure the activity is not viewed as punishment

- Family time- adopt a lifestyle that includes regular physical activity of all family members: walk after dinner, games that incorporate movement.

At school-

School health programme--

- Set Nutrition Education Goals –encourage students to make lifelong healthy food choices. Establish nutrition standards for all food available in school setting.**School snacks should be changed to whole grains, baked not fried snacks.** Healthy snacks (fruit tray, finger sandwiches, cheese cubes & crackers) should be provided with proper portion size at canteen counter. Also,**vending machines should be removed from within schools.**

- Set Physical Activity Goals to promote wellness – help students to understand the short and long term benefits of a physically active & healthy lifestyle. In pre-primary and primary section; celebrations should be in non-food way (active game chosen by students, special art project etc). Schools should also provide an environment that fosters this behaviour. Praising, Recognising, privileging and encouraging is essential.A School can increase physical activities by setting a walking club for staff and or students, teaching academics through physical activity, Keeping kids active at recess. Promotion of lifestyle physical activities to students & staff can be a good option.

- Teenagers weight Balance
- Regular meals with non elimination of breakfast is prime requisite. Insistance on consumption of vegetables, complex carbs, fiber and decreasing consumption of fast food and basic sugars.

Social awareness--

1. We need to encourage and praise Food Services for the healthy changes.

4. Advertisements trick children's taste buds and wrapping affects their preferences

Even carrots, milk, and apple juice taste better to the children when they are wrapped nicely.

CHAPTER 8

FEMALE OBESITY

The major factors that contribute to a person's ideal weight are Height, Gender, Age, Body frame, Body type. Female obesity brings alongwith it many related physical and psychological problems that affect women and th way they perceive themselves.

Types of female obesity-
Type I-BMI-30-34.9

Simple obesity- constitutional and acquired.

Constitutional- from infancy. Non-sensitive to insulin. Poor cure effect.

Acquired- diet induced. Early adult onset. Weight increases on limbs mainly.

Secondary obesity- disease associated.

Hypothalamic, metabolic, cushing's, PCOS, insulin tumour, hypothyroid.

Prevalence
National family health survey (NFHS-2) in 1998-1999, 2005-2006
Prevalence of obesity among Indian women has elevated from 0.6% to 12.6% (increased by 24.52%)
Prevalence is more profound in women of age 40-49 yrs. (23.7%)

Residing in cities (23.5%)

Having high qualification (23.8%)

Highest wealth quintile (30.5%)

Total prevalence has increased by 15% in last decade.
Obesity and Hormones-

GH levels in obese people are lower than in normal weight oestrogens (from ovaries) and androgens(from testes) decide body fat distribution.

In older age group, these hormones get reduced, then main site of oetrogen production becomes fat in menopausal women.

Women of child bearing age store fat in lower body (pear shape).

 Old male and post menopausal females tend to store fat around abdomen (apple shape).

Lack of oestrogen leads to excessive weight gain.

Excess adiposity during childhood may advance puberty in girls and delay puberty in boys.

Female are more prone than male to obesity. This sexual dimorphism is due to plasma leptin concentration.

 Inceasing BMI ----   % of oligomenorrhoea increases from 18% to 32%.

% of amenorrhoea increases from 2% to 13%

% of anovulation increases from 32% to 55%

Scanty and infrequent menstruation is treated by hormonal therapy that may lead to obesity.

Obesity and Artavkshaya and Hormonal Imbalance-

Increased level of Free fatty acids (FFA) due to large measure to the presence of more lipolytically active intra-abdominal adipocytes.

Increased level of FFA is associated with inhibition of hepatic clearance of insulin and thus with increased insulinism and its consequences.

Levels of basal and stimulated levels of norepinephrine are increased in obesity.

Obesity predisposes to carbohydrate intolerance by increasing insulin resistance.

Serum testosterone level increases in obese woman and this hyperandrogenaemia is responsible for irregular menses and hirsuitism.

Obesity especially **intra-abdominal adiposity** is associated with increased free fatty acid (FFA) concentration in plasma which exercises major negative effect on insulin sensitivity in both muscle and liver. Besides insulin resistance, both lipotoxicity and glucotoxicity may initiate and enable a vicious circle dependable for metabolic impairment.

Fat content accumulated in women is twice the amount found in men of the same age.**Body and mental changes during puberty, pregnancy or menopause can lead to obesity.**

Pathogenesis

Obesity is associated with 3 biochemical alterations that affect normal ovulation

1. Hyperinsulinaemia
2. Increased Peripheral Conversion Of Androgen To Estrogen
3. Decreased Level Of Sex Hormone Binding Globulin (SHBG) Resulting In Increased Level Of Free Oestradiol And Testosterone.

SHBG tends to linearly decrease with increasing body fat and may lead to increase in fraction of free Androgens and thus Estrogen level decreases. SHBG levels are regulated by complex of factor including Estrogen, Iodothyronies and Growth hormone as stimulating agents and Androgens and Insulin as inhibiting factor.

The net balance of this regulation with dominant role of Insulin which inhibits SHBG. Synthesis in liver may be responsible for decrease of SHBG concentration observed in obesity.

Fat represent a site of intense sex hormone metabolism and interconversion due to presence of several steroidogenetic enzymes such as 3 beta dehydrogenese, 17 betahydroxydehydrogenase and aromatase systems.

Obesity may thus add further specific mechanism in the development of androgen excess in women and decreases oestrogen.

Treatment

Anti obesity drugs act as anti-metabolites, capable of blocking pathway of oxidation of fatty acids. They alter either appetite, metabolism or absorption of calories.

Mechanism of drugs-

Decrease lipid absorption

Decrease energy intake

Decrease pre-adipocyte differentiation and proliferation

Decrease lipogenesis and increase lipolysis.

Modulation of carbohydrate metabolism

Increase satiety

Block dietary fat absorption

Increase energy Expenditure

Increase water elimination

Enhance mood

Female Obesity Control Programme-

- To identify the obesity rates for adolescent girls between the ages of 13 -19 years.
- To explain the factors associated with obesity and overweight of children and adolescents
- To describe various program models for nutrition and physical activity programs
- To recommend collaborators and resources at the state and local levels for nutrition and physical activity programs

Special Treatment Plans For Females

Combination of therapies as well as **Combination of drugs** changes as per age, stage (Puberty, Child bearing age, Menopause) constitution,physical built, psychology, occupation, with associated diseases and complications of obesity.

- Pre pubertal stage
- Fertile Female
- Post partum stage
- Postmenopausal stage
- Obesity with DM, HT, Hypothyroidism, cardiac problems , PCOD etc.

CHAPTER 9

MANAGEMENT OF OBESITY - AYURVEDIC VIEW

Sthoola is considered as Nindita. Management of Sthoulya is difficult as long term, consistent, troublesome treatment alongwith liestyle modification with diet and exercise is mandatory. Need of the hour is to treat rationally so that complications can be reduced or prevented. In this regard approach of Ayurveda is more safe, comprehensive and rational.

Ayurvedic View-
- Ayurvedic approach in achieving ideal weight, is based on taking a **realistic look at our body type** and then nourishing it back to natural health. It is about getting to know your body and becoming in tune with its rhythm.
- **Permanent resetting of mind- body's ability to regulate itself by calming nervous system, enhancing digestive fires and regulating storage of energy and fat is done.**
- In ayurveda, rather than universal approach to solving problems, it is always **patient specific**, towards all diseases and obesity in particular. Strategies are designed for each person after a careful analysis of condition of person's body, mind, soul, dosha status and constitution.
- Lifestyle modification as per constitution is advised especially regarding diet and exercise.
- Increase in intake of foods that enhance digestive fire like ginger, bitter melons, dark bitter greens etc. is advised.

Elimination of Ama—
- Ama is byproduct of inefficient or incomplete digestion. It tends to clog up circulatory, lymph and other channels of body. Getting rid of ama is primary strategy.

- It's highly impossible to treat any imbalance of physiology when ama is present and it is extremely difficult, perhaps impossible to lose weight This is why so many people who have limited their diets to the point of virtual starvation still have failed to accomplish their goals. So, it's essential to take practical steps to eliminate ama in order to lose weight and keep it off permanently. ama is, quite simply, a key in the pathogenesis of obesity.
- Sipping of warm water processed with powders of dry ginger, khus, and Musta.
- Turmeric + Triphala+ Trikatu +Honey with warm water.

For two types of therapies are to be formulated for treating the over-obese (atisthula) and over-lean (atikrsa) persons. In general, for reducing the bulk of the obese (sthulanam karsanam parti). heavy (guru) and non-saturating (atarpanam) while for promoting the bulk of the lean (krsanam brnhanrtham), light (laghu) and saturating therapy (santarpana) is prescribed.

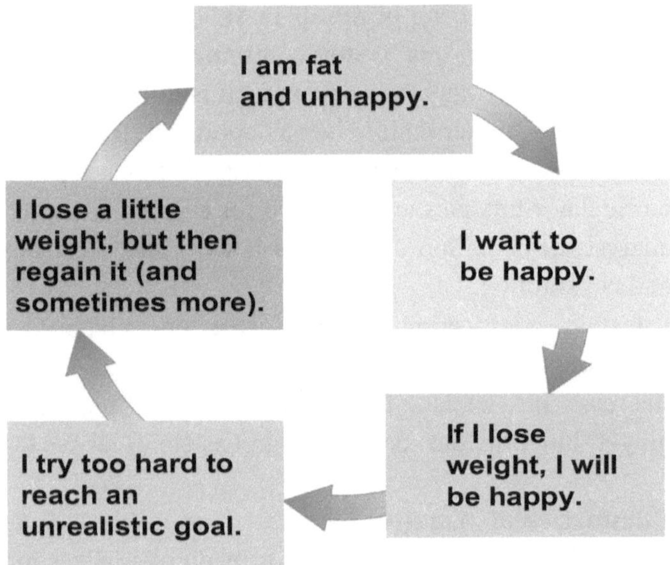

TREATMENT PLAN FOR OBESITY

- ❖ Nidanasya Parivarjarna – Find And Nullify Cause
- ❖ Satata Karshana Chikitsa – Continuous/ Repeated/ Periodic Treatment
- ❖ Guru Apatarpana Ahar- Diet Regulation
- ❖ Langhana Chikitsa
- ❖ Shodhana Rupi Langhana - Panchkarma
- ❖ Shamana Rupi Langhan- Pharmacotherapy
- ❖ Pathyapathya – Do's And Don'ts

BMI is one of the criterion for designing treatment plan.

BMI	PLAN OF TREATMENT
25-26.9	Drug, Diet (Pathyapathya), Exercise, Behaviour Therapy
27-29.9	Panchkarma followed by Drug, Diet (Pathyapathya), Exercise, Lifestyle modification
30-34.9	Repeated, periodic Panchkarma alongwith long term pharmacotherapy, Continuous (Permanent) Diet control, Exercise, Lifestyle modification
35 AND ABOVE	Surgery, Panchkarma Pre and Post surgery AND continued periodically alongwith long term pharmacotherapy, Continuous (Permanent) Diet control, Exercise, Lifestyle modification

Shodhan Chikitsa

PANCHKARMA therapy should be done as **Primary Treatment** for

-Heredity of obesity

-Genetically obese

-Repeated weight gain after weight loss

-Lifestyle Disorder

-Physically unfit for vigorous exercise

-Need of speedy weight loss for some reason

PLAN OF TREATMENT
1. Shodhan Chikitsa-Purificatory Measures-PANCHKARMA

AIM- To remove accumulated toxins out of body
- To cleanse channels to facilitate circulation of nutrients
- To increase body's receptibility for drugs and diet
- To modify, improve Digestion and Metabolism

PANCHKARMA – 5 FOLD THERAPY

Panchkarma therapies advocated before pharmacotherapy and other treatments give better, fast and long standing results in obesity management. Out of 5, three are proved to be more beneficial for Obesity Vaman , Virechan, Basti. Swedan and Udvartan also play a major role in treatment.

- **Vaman** (medicated vomitting)
- **Virechana** (medicated purgation)
- **Basti** (enema therapy)-particularly Lekhan Basti.Herbs used in basti- Ushakadi
- **Raktamokshana**-Blood letting therapy

Other useful purificatory measures are-
- **Dhumpan**-medicated smoking
- **Swedan**- Sudation therapy-
    Kuti Sweda, Ruksha sweda, Anagni sweda
- **Udvartana**-herbal powder massage-
    Rubbing of dry powders with or without friction is helpful especially for fat deposits at subcutaneous level.
    Herbs   for   Udvartana-Triphala,musta,   Neem,   Haridra, Daruharidra, Tulasi, Ashwagandha, Musterd, Lodhra, Vacha

Out of various Basti , **Lekhan, Vaitaran, Ardhamatrik, Yog Basti** are more beneficial.

LEKHAN BASTI

- Enema that contains drugs that are having LIPOLYSING capacity.
- ENEMA IS GIVEN ON ALTERNATE FORTNIGHTS FOR 3 CYCLES.
- Combination contains-

1st combination-300 - 400 ml of Decoction of herbs (Musta, Kushtha, Haridra, Daruharidra,Vacha, Chitrak, Karanj, Hemavati, Varun, Vidanga)Kutaki, Ativisha mixed with 100 ml of cow urine, 80 ml of honey, 10 gm of saindhav and 5 gm of yavakshar.

2nd combination-300-400 ml decoction of Triphala 10 gm of powder of Ushak, Saindhav Shilajatu, Kasis, Hing, Tuttha and Moorchchita sarshap oil mixed with 100 ml of cow urine, 80 ml of honey, 5 gm of yavakshar.

PANCHKARMA- Maadhutailika Basti

'Maadhutailika Basti', a type of 'Aasthaapana Basti' also termed as 'Niruha Basti' is a mixture of oil, honey, 'kwaatha' (decoction) and 'Kalka' (fine paste obtained after wet grinding of the plant material). These ingredients are immiscible with each other. A homogenous mixture is required for actual administration of 'Basti'.
Simlarly, Triphaladi Tail / Mahasugandhi Tail can be used for Basti.
Ingredient of Maadhutailika Basti -

1. *Ricinus communis Linn.* (*Erand moola*) roots.

2. *Foenicum vulgare Mill.* (*Shatapushpa*) fruits (Fennel).

3. *Randia spinosa* poir (*Madanphal*) seeds (Emetic nut).

4. Honey.

5. Sesame Oil.

6. Rock Salt.

7. Potable water.

Exrernal treatment

- **Udvartan-** Retrograde powder massage by rubbing(with pressure). Drugs used are having penetrating, scraping capacity. e.g.- Powders of Triphala, Nimb, Nagarmotha, Vacha, Shunthee, Agaru, Haridra, Daruharidra, Shirish, Khus, Lodhra, Nagkeshar, Arkapatra kshar, White clay,Ash of cow dunk
- Lepa- Local application of medicated paste
- Snehan and Mardan- Oil application with variable pressure and in direction from distal to proximal end.
- Swedan- Sudation especially Kutiswed.
- Snehan and Swedan should be done before advocating Panchkarma Therapies.

- **Drugs and technique of therapy are equally important.**
- **All applications should be from distal to proximal end.**

2. Shaman Chikitsa

These are pacificatory measures that are advocated generally after purificatory procedures.

AIM-
- To pacify vitiated dosha responsible for existing obesity
- To tone up fat by removal (lekhan- scraping) of abnormal, excess fat from areas where it has got accumulated in abundance.
- therapy with herbs, diet, exercises and lifestyle .
- Use of Bitter, pungent astringent taste
- Drugs of Dry, hot, sharp, scraping qualities
- Anupan- luke warm water and honey

Dhatutarpan chikitsa-

Refers to providing adequate nourishment to make you feel satisfied but not in excess to be stored as fat.

Agnimandyahara chikitsa –

Improves Digestion and Metabolism.

Apunarbhav Chikitsa-

Measures those are undertaken to avoid regain of lost weight, maintainance of health and healthy weight toning up of body constituents. so, not to allow fat to accumulate within lax tissues.

Drugs For Obesity

Especially for **Abdominal Obesity-**

- Lauha rasayan, lohasav, loharishta
- Varunadi kwath
- Chitrak, kutaki, trikatu combination.
- Musta+ Shunthee Jal
- ½ tsp honey + ½ tsp basil leaves - paste in 1 glass of luke warm water to drink.
- 1 glass of water + soak 2 tablespoon of horse gram & keep it for a day. -Drink early morning on empty stomach.
- Arogyavardhini,Chandraprabha,Punarnava mandur, gomutra haritaki,Medohar guggulu, navak guggul,Trivang bhasma.

To reduce fat and for getting relief from obesity-one should follow certain measures, for instance:

i) Upavasa (fasting and dieting or abandoning food-abstinence from heavy cereals and edible in high quantity and high calories or much nourishing food etc.).

An obese person should always use following cereals and food articles as well as suitable measures:

purana Sali (old-not freshly harvested rice esp; Sali), Mudga, Kulattha, Uddalaka (vankodrava), Kodrava.

ii) Asukha shayya (sleeping on uncomfortable bed or avoiding luxurious, highly comfortable bed using modern amenities for making it softer and bulky etc.)

iii) Sattvoudarya (psychic generosity and courtesy);

iv)   Tamojaya (countering sleep and adverse effects and characteristics of temoguna)

The obesity caused by santarpana (saturation) should be checked by following measures :

As obese person who is inclined to practice these measures as his favorites and prefers to consume yava (barley) and shyamaka cereals as food articles, definitely succeeds in getting rid of obesity.

Dhumapana (medicated smoking), krodha (anger) and raktamoksana (blood letting) are beneficial to obese condition. After digestion of food once ingested, one should use barley (yava) and wheat (godhuma) regularly for food preparations which should be consumed by patient in routine diet.

CHAPTER 10

STHAULYA CHIKITSA
- AYURVEDIC DRUGS AND FORMULATIONS

Triphala - Sharangadhara Samhita, 2, 2, 118

It is combination of 3 healings herb, their fruits are used.

* **Amalaki (emblica officinalis),-**
* **Haritaki (terminalia chebula)**
* **Bibhitaki (terminalia belerica)**

Triphala (triad of fruit-drugs consisting Haritaki, Bibhitaka And Amalaki), cooked in water for preparing a decoction which is mixed with honey. It is orally given in persons suffering from obesity (medoroga).

Triphala powder with honey or lukewarm water mixed with honey is taken in obesity (medoroga).

Oral administration of butter milk (takra) and Nimba, rough food (ruksanna), drink (pana), cow's urine and Triphala is medicine for the disorder of lipid metabolism (snehavyapati bheshajam).

Diseases caused by saturation (santartpana) like prameha, medoroga (obesity) etc. are alleviated by the administration of butter milk (takra) with haritaki (abhaya), triphala (triad group of three fruit drugs viz. haritaki, bibhltaka and amalaki) and arishta (fermented liquors).

Powder of Triphala and Trikatu is mixed with oil and salt (satailam lavananvitam). This recipe is recommended for internal use, regularly for six months. It is effective in alleviating aggravated Kapha and Vata, and it reduces fat (medapaham).

Effects of Triphala - all dosha balancing, very good cleanser ,purifies blood rejuvenating herb. it decreases excessive Meda

reduces serum cholesterol, reduces the plaque formation in the arteries ,high blood pressure, provides remarkable protection in CVD, In a study conducted by the American Botanical Council, it was shown that Triphala greatly reduced blood glucose levels in diabetic rats .

In Triphala, main anti obesity action is because of Haritaki.

Pathya-Haritaki

(a)   The powder of Haritaki is mixed with honey; it is taken with sura after mixing honey in early *morning* . It is useful in checking perspiration and providing pleasant odour in obese body.

(b)   Paste *of Haritaki fruits should be anointed on body of obese and bathed thereafter.* It is useful to check perspiration in obesity.

(c)   Equal parts of Bilva and Haritaki is pounded for preparing a paste. It is extremely applied to check bad odour.

Haritaki (fruits) is recommended as most effective drug for alleviating diseases caused by saturation (santarpanajanita rogah). There are various ailing conditions which are produced due to saturating foods or diets, drinks etc. (ahara) as well as conducts or physical activities (vihara). Among such diseases, medoroga (obesity) is an important disease, and the drug haritaki is one of the major medicines.

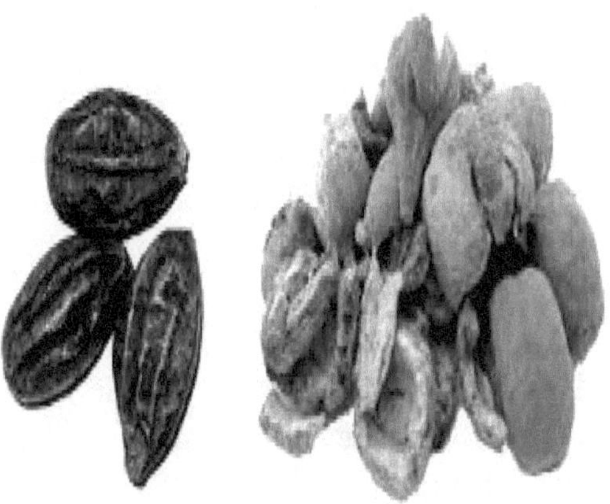

Guggulu- (Commiphora mukul) - Bhavaprakasa, madhya. 39,30
- Light, dry, sharp, subtle, mobile, non slimy
- T-bitter, pungent,   A-Hot, PE- Pungent

- All dosha balancing –by Prabhav
- Useful part = Resin   Old guggulu- scraping quality
- It is strong detoxifying and cleansing and rejuvenating herb.
- Lower cholesterol and triglycerides and maintain or improve HDL/LDL ratio, anti-inflammatory effects.
- There is prescription of 'Navaka Guggulu' which is recommended for oral administration in medoroga (obesity) and anomalies caused by aggravation of vata and kapha doshas.
- Pharmaco-dynamics and therapeutic efficacy of Guggulu have been described in various treaties. Medicinal effects notably include anti-obesity property of Guggulu.
- Guggulu has both kinds of medicinal utilities-fresh (nava) guggulu acts as aphrodisiac and nourishing, while old (purana) is efficacious as apakarshana medicine.
- An obese person is advised to use regularly Shilajatu, Guggulu and other various drugs and cereals etc. for reducing fat.
- Rasanjana, Brihat Panchamula, Guggulu, Shilajatu and Agnimantha should be mixed. It is given in obesity (medoroga).
- Purified Guggulu is given with cow urine , which is useful in obesity and ailments like oedema, anaemia and udararoga. Similarly the decotion of Punarnava, Devadaru, Haritaki and Guduchi.
- Guggulu (shuddha) is taken with cow urine, with decoction of Brihat Panchamula or Agnimantha. It is prescribed in treatment of obesity.

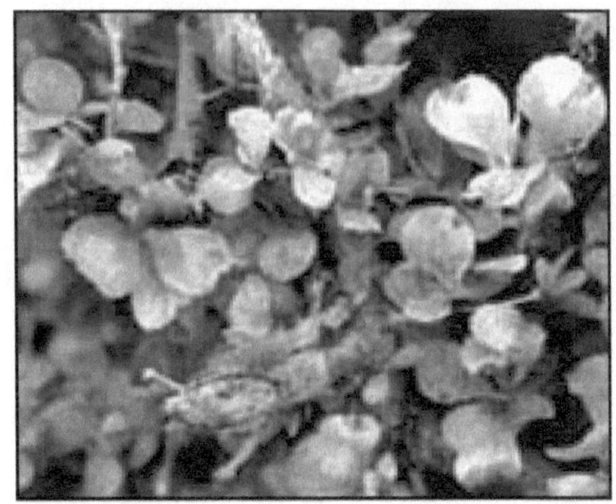

Vidanga –Embelia ribes

- Light dry sharp   T- pungent ,astringent
- A- hot   PE-pungent
- consists of dried mature fruits of Embelia ribes Burm. f. (Fam.Myrsinaceae), large scandent shrub .
- Vata kapha pacifying, agni stimulating,
- Vidanga allays vata, it is diuretic, a mild purgative and kills worms, it is an appetizer, digestive, blood purifier and rejuvenator.

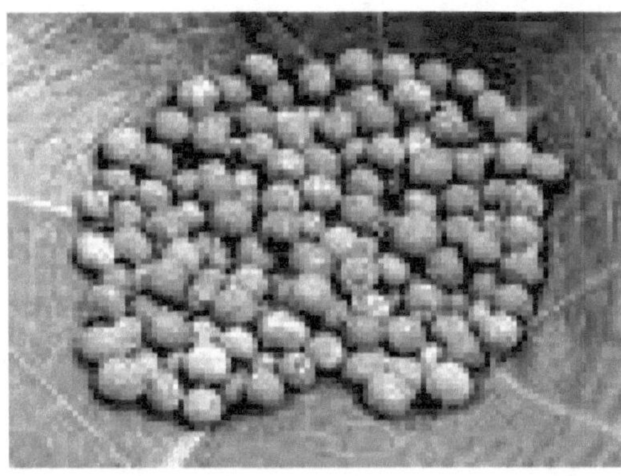

Shilajatu-Mineral pitch

- It is the resins that oozes out from Himalayan Mountains

- Light dry   T-bitter pungent astringent
- A- hot   scraping quality
- Mainly Vata and Kapha balancing
- It decreases excessive fat, very helpful in enhancing sexual powers. It is anti inflammatory and antioxidant

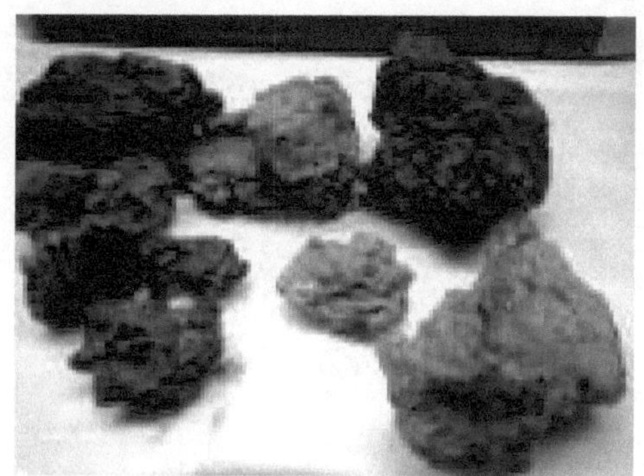

Nagarmotha (Cyperus rotundus)

Nagarmotha is the herb which has been described in Ayurveda as the best ama-pachaka or corrective and remover of endo-toxins.

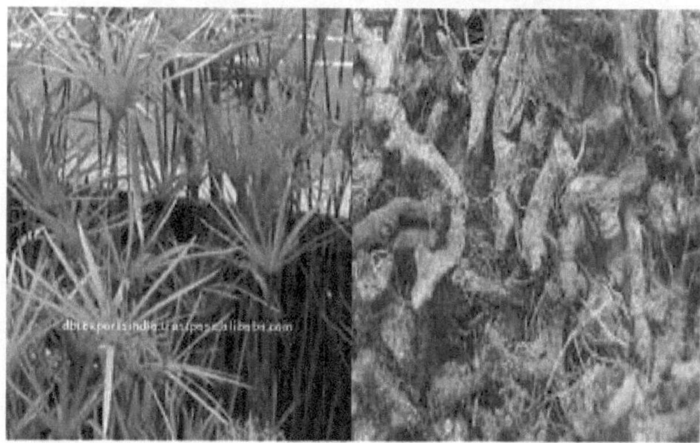

Chitraka

Chitraka consists of dried mature root of Plumbago zeylanica Linn. (Fam.
Plumbaginaceae) , a large perennial sub-scandent shrub.

- Vangasena, in Medoroga, 22 states that the root of Chitraka-in powder or any other form-should be used in Sthoulya chikitsa.

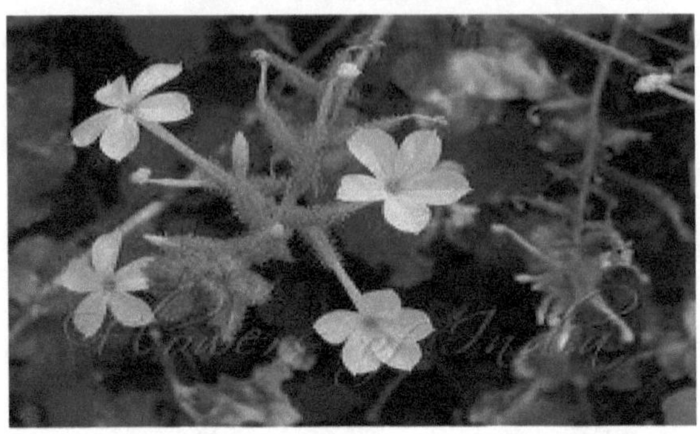

Shunthee

Consists of dried rhizome of Zingiber officinale Roxb.
(Fam.Zinglberaceae), widely cultivated in India, rhizomes
 dug in January-February, buds and roots removed,
soaked overnight-in water, decorticated, and some times treated with lime and dried.

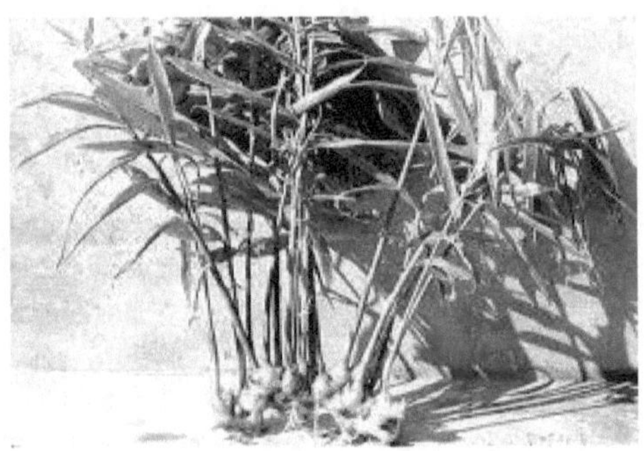

Maricha (Black pepper)
Batanical Name: *Piper nigrum*

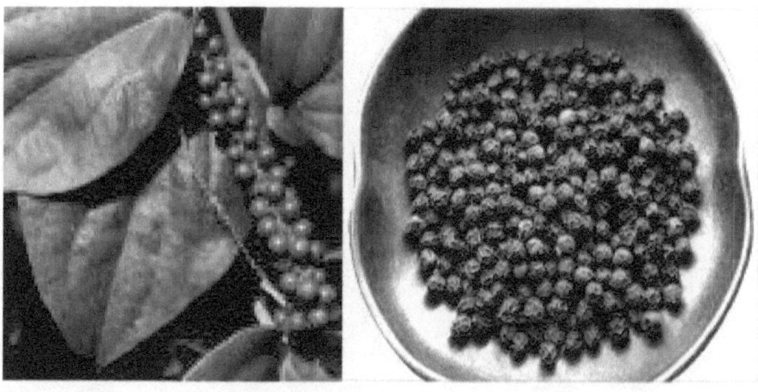

Pippali (Fruit)

Pippali consists of the dried, immature, catkin-like fruits with bracts of Piper

longum Linn. (Fam. Piperaceae), a slender, aromatic climber

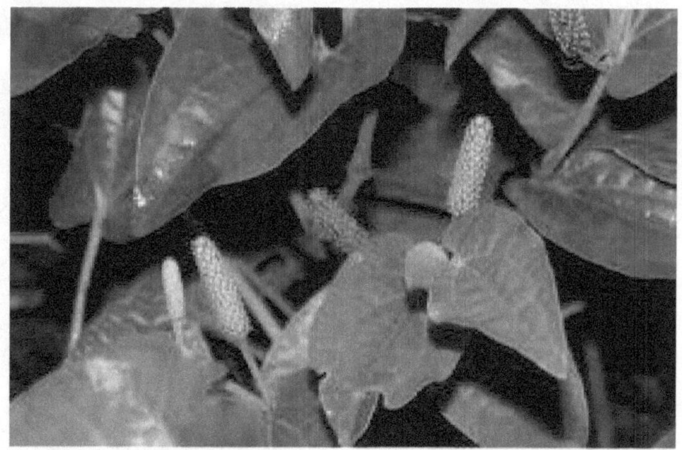

Devdaru (Heart Wood)

Devad¡ru consists of dried heart wood of Cedrus deodara (Roxb.) Loud. (Fam.

Pinaceae), a very large and tall ever green tree

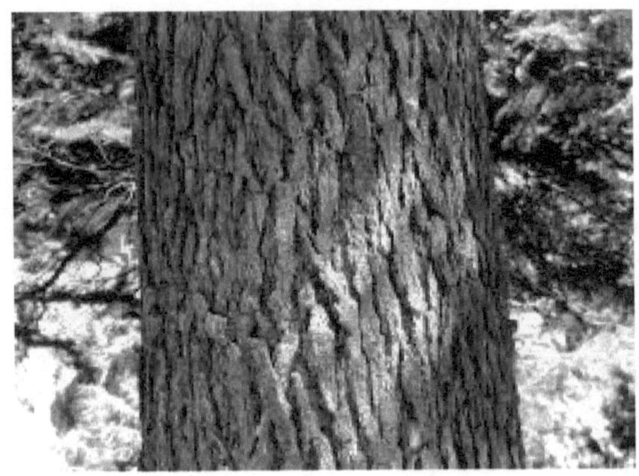

Atasi

Atasi consists of dried, ripe seeds of Linum usitatissimum Linn. (Fam. Linaceae),

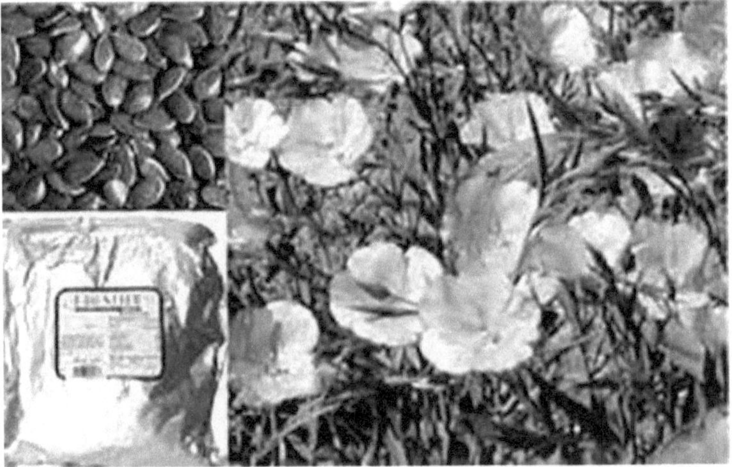

Kanchanar

Kanchanara consists of the dried, stem bark of Bauhinia variegata Blume (Fam.
Leguminosae):

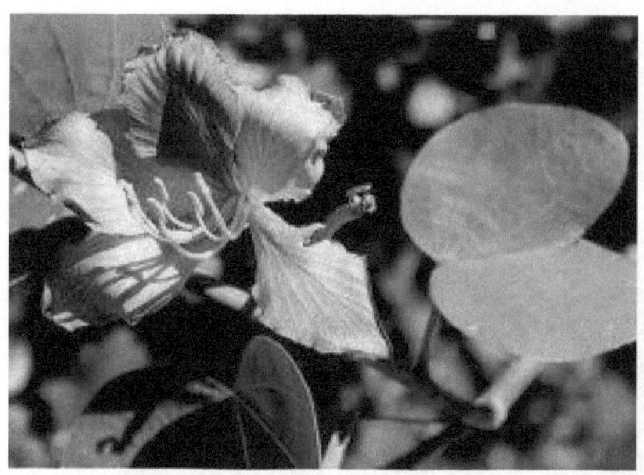

Tvak

Tvak is the dried inner bark (devoid of cork and cortex) of the coppiced shoots of
stem of Cinnamomum zeylanicum Blume. (Fam. Lauraceae),

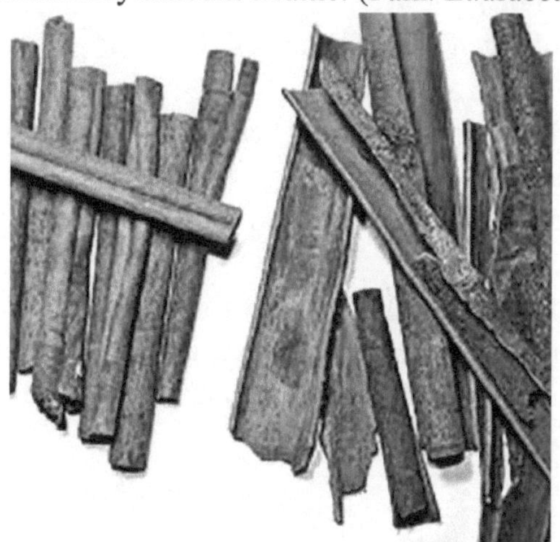

Tvakpatra

Tvakpatra consists of dried mature leaves of Cinnamomum tamala (Buch. Ham.)
Nees & Eberm. (Fam. Lauraceae):
External application in the form of anointment of Patra, Balaka, Aguru, Ushira And Chandana is recommended in obesity for checking foul smell of the body. (Vaidya Manorama, 16, 137)

Flowers of Brihati are applied in the specific process (as given in text) on medovikarajanya kotha.

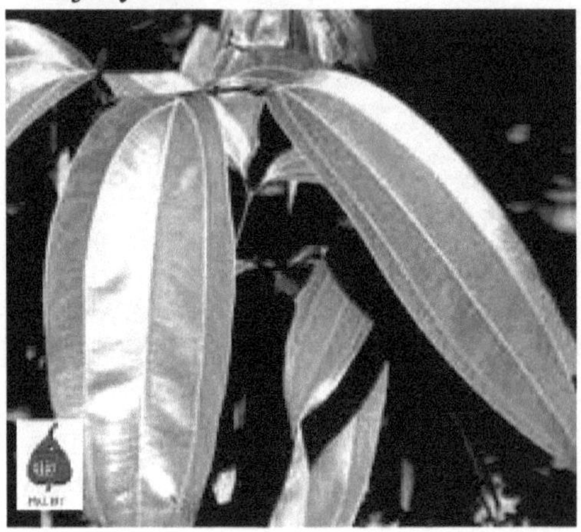

Yava (Whole Plant)

Yava consists of dried whole plant of Hordeum vulgare Linn. Syn. H. sativum Pers.

(Fam. Poaceae), an annual, erect, herb, 50 to 100 cm high, cultivated chiefly in North

India, for its de husked fruits known as Barley in trade . Charaka Samhita, sutra. 21, 23

States that Powder (flour) of Yava (barley) should be mixed. It is recommended for use regularly. It is suggested as an excellent remedy for alleviating medoroga (obesity). Shyamaka and Yava are wholesome diet for obese persons.

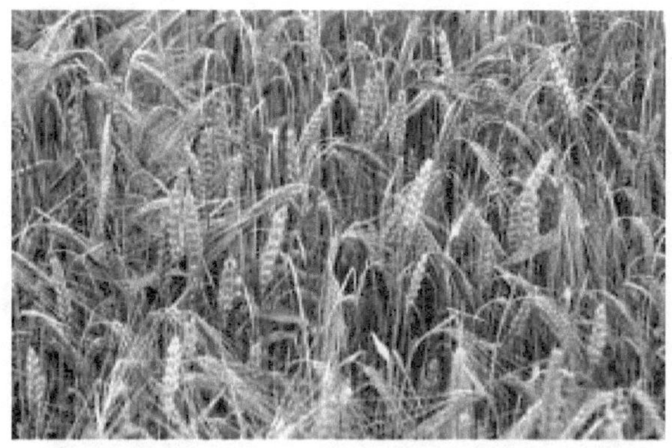

Yavakshara

It is an alkaline preparation made with the ingredient in the Formulation composition given below.

Formulation composition:

1. Yava (API) Bhasma *Hordeum vulgare* Pl. 1 part
2. Jala API Water 6 parts

Dose: ½ to 1 g daily in divided dose.

Anupāna: Warm water, Gh"ta

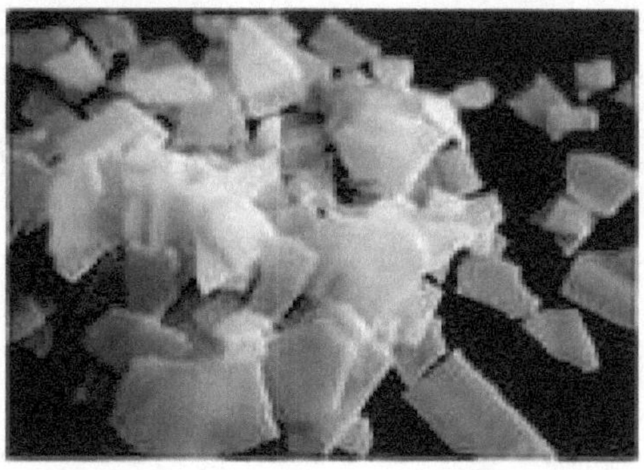

Kukkutanakhee

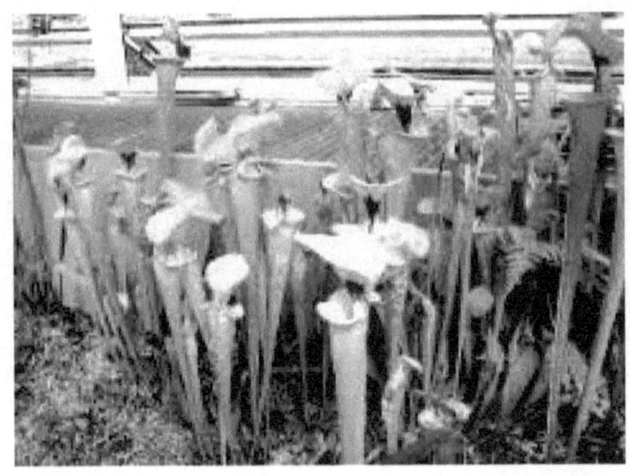

Agnimantha

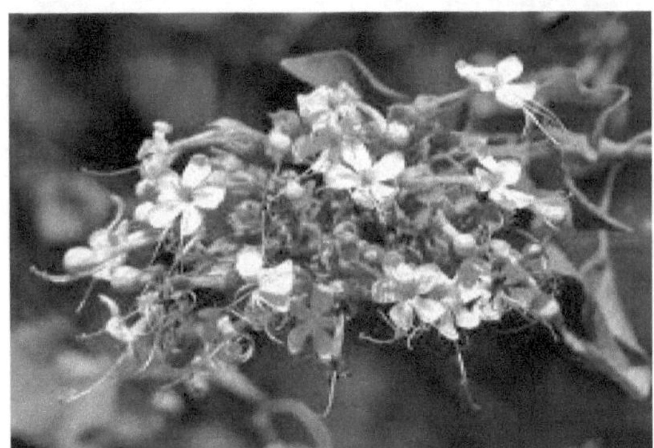

Agnimantha - Charaka Samhita, sutra. 21, 24

Decoction (or expressed juice) of agnimantha is recommended as an effective remedy for medoroga (obesity).

Honey

- It promotes health and digestion.
- It is a powerful antioxidant.
- Honey pacifies digestive fire.
- Regulates increased appetite to normal
- Though sweet in taste, it has good scraping action that reduces fat.

- Different varieties of honey have specific effect on various diseases
- Honey acts as catalyst. As and when mixed with different drugs, will potentiate and hasten their action.
- Some formulations for obesity—
- Honey + ginger mixed in equal quantity and taken 3 gm.before food
- Triphala powder/ decoction + honey– for 6 months

Gomutra

- Cow urine is beneficial as it:
- Lowers the levels of cholesterol
- Improves liver function.
- Slows down the process of aging
- Gives strength to brain and heart
- Destroys the toxic effects of medicinal residues in the body

Rasanjanam - Astahga Hrdaya, 40, 49.

(a) Rasanjana (semi-solid extract of Darvi) is considered to be a best medicine for obesity

(b) Rasanjana is one of the useful drugs which are recommanded for administering in treatment of obesity.

Bilva - Sharngadhara Samhita, 2, 2, 11

a) For checking bad odour from obese body, the juice bilva leaves is considered to be useful in condition of obesity.

b) The decoction of Brihat Panchamula (consisting of a group of five drugs viz. Bilva, Agnimantha, Shyonaka, Kashmari and Patala) is prepared and same is mixed with honey. It is given orally to obese person for alleviation of obesity (medoroga).

c) A paste of Bilva and Haritaki (combining in equal parts) should be applied over obese body.

Urubuka-Eranda

The root of eranda smeared with honey is kept over night in water. This water (extract) is orally given in obese person, especially for reducing enlarged abdomen (jatharavrddhi).

It is prescribed for internal use by obese person who is to consume wholesome diet during the course of medication.

Kshara of Eranda patra is prepared and it is mixed with Hingu (asafoetida). This mixture is prescribed for intake by obese person. Patient should depend on rice diet. It alleviates obesity in condition of excessive fat.

Chincha -Bhavaprakasa, Madhyama. 39, 72

Juice of chincha leaves is useful for external application on body of obese persons. It alleviates bad odour.

Babbula - *Bhavaprakasa, Sthulya. 39, 78-79*

Leaves of babbula are prescribed in *obesity. The* human body should be anointed with the paste of babbula leaves and then with the paste of haritakl fruits. Afterwards , patient should take bath in water prepared of these two kinds of paste (prepared in water). excessive perspiration is checked in obese persons.

Guduchi - Chikitsa Kalika, 319

Decoction (or any other form) of Guduchi is useful in obesity and other diseases (e.g. Vatarakta, Shlipada, Halimaka, Pandu and Kamala).

Badari - Chakradatta, 36, 16

The paste prepared of badari leaves is mixed with liquid gruel and sour gruel is administered. It alleviates obesity.

Bhurja - Bhavaprakasa, Vatadivarga 47-48

Medicinal properties of bhurja are described and medicinal efficiency of drug bhurja against obesity (medoroga) is highlighted in Nighantu.

Salasaradigana - Susruta Samhita, cikitsa. 18, 53

Powder of drugs belonging to salasaradigana is mixed in cow urine (gomutra) is to be given in morning. It is useful in galaganda caused by fat (medovikarajanya goitre).

Bijaka - Vaidya *Manorama, 12,30*
One should take seasame oil in the morning or decoction of the heartwood of asana (bijaka) mixed with honey, it alleviates obesity, especially useful for very obese person (atisthula).

Surana - Vaidya Manorama, 16, 139.

Mature tuber of surana is pounded with Shunthi and water. This paste is applied on cyst-medogranthi.

Atimuktaka-Madhavi - Bhavaprakasa, cikitsa, 39, 24.

The seed-kernel (bijamadhyam) should be taken/ licked with honey; it is effective to check the growth of abdomen due to obesity, in persons having fat belly.

Root of Madhavi is taken with butter milk in obesity. It is specifically useful for slimming the waist.

Gavedhuka - Bhavaprakasa, Chikitsa. 39, 22

Gruel is made of the parched grains of Gavedhuka and it is mixed with honey. This remedy is considered to be useful in reducing bulk of the obese body.

Flour of parched grains of gavedhuka and barley (yava) are mixed for preparing 'saktu'. It is given to obese persons .

Haridra - Bhavaprakasa, Sthoulya. 39, 72

Roasted pieces of Haridra are ground for preparing a powder. It is applied on body as 'udvartana' which counters foul odour of obese.

Jambu - Bhavaprakasha, Sthoulya, 39, 76

Decoction of Jambu is useful as angaraga in obesity (medoroga).

Patola - Bhavaprakasha, Sthoulya. 39, 20
Decoction of Patola (leaves) and Chitraka (root) is prepared and it is mixed with Shatapushpa and Hingu. This mixture is taken by obese person. It is useful in reducing excess fat.

Tambula - Vaidya Manorama, 12, 31
A betel leaf mixed with 10 gm of Maricha (fruits), is taken orally with cold water . This yog is suggested for use regularly for two months. It makes highly obese person quite lean and thin.

Shakhotaka - Sharangadhara Samhita, 2, 2, 127
Decoction of bark obtained from tree of Shakhotaka should be prepared and it is to be mixed with cow's urine. It should be taken by patient of Shleepada and medodosha.

Shyamaka - Vrindamadhava, 36.4
The regular consumption of specific wholesome diet combining Yava and Shyamaka is recommended in obesity (medoroga). It is quite helpful to alleviate excessive fat.

Mundi -Alambusha - Bhavaprakasha, Chikitsa. 39, 70

Goups Of Drugs Advised By Sushruta
1. Salsaradi Gana
2. Varunadi Gana
3. Lodhradi Gana
4. Arkadi Gana
5. Mushkakadi Gana
6. Ooshakadi Gana
7. Vallipanchamoola/ Kantakpanchamoola
8. Kaphasanshamana Gana

Herbal Drugs useful in Obesity

Sr. No.	Name of Herb	Latin name	Useful Part
1	Agnimantha	Clerodendrum Phlomidis Linn.	Root, root bark, Bark, leaves
2	Bhurja	Betula utilis D. Don.	Bark
3	Paribhadra	Erythrina Indica Lam	Roots
4	Parisha	Thespesia populnea S. ex C.	Bark, roots
5	Patola	Trichosanthes dioica Roxb.	Fruits, Leaves
6	Pushkaramula	Inula racemosa Hook. F. J.	Root
7	Varuna	Crataeva religiosa Buch-Ham	Bark, roots
8	Vasa	Adhotoda vasica Nees	Roots, Leaves
9	Yava	Hordeum vulgare Linn	Barley (Fruits)
10	Shigru	Moringa olifera Lam	Roots, Bark,,Seeds
11	Chitraka	Plumbago zeylanica Linn	Root
12	Eranda	Ricinus communis Linn.	Root
13	Guggulu	Comiphora mukul (H.ex.S.)	Resin
14	Haridra	Curcum longa Linn	Rhizome
15	Haritaki	Terminalila chebula Retz	Fruits
16	Chincha	Tamarindus indica Linn	Fruits

17	Babbula	Acacia Arabica wild	Bark, other parts
18	Badari	Zizyphus jujube Lam	Fruit, Root
19	Bijaka	Pterocarpus marsupium Roxb	Wood
20	Bilva	Aegle marmelos Corr.	Leaves, Bark, Roots
21	Jambu	Syzygium cumini (Linn)	Fruit-rind Skeels
22	Gavedhuka	Coix lachrymal-jobi	Seeds (grains)
23	Shirisha	Albizzia-lebbeck Benth.	Bark, seeds
24	Tambula Nagavalli	Piper betle Linn.	Leaves
25	Yava	Hordeum vulgare Linn	Grains (seeds)
26	Shakhotaka	Streblus asper Lour	Bark
27	Hingu	Ferula narthex Boiss	Exudate (resin)
28	Mustaka	Cyperus rotundus Linn	Root
29	Vidanga	Embelia ribes Burm. F.	Fruits
30	Rasanjana-Daruharidra	Berberis aristata DC	Root, Wood
31	Devadaru	Cedrus deodara (Roxb.)	Heartwood
32	Syonaka	Oxoxylon indica Vent.	Bark, Root
33	Patala	StereospermumSua veolens DC	Bark, Root
34	Kasmari	Gmelina asborea Roxb.	Bark, Root

35	Mudga	Vigna radiate (Linn.)	Grains (Seeds)
36	Karavellaka	Momordia charantia Linn	Fruits
37	Methika	Trigonella foenum-graceum Linn	Seeds
38	Ardraka-Shunthi	Zingiber officinale Roxb.	Rhizome
39	Pippali	Piper longum Linn	Fruits
40	Maricha	Piper nigrum Linn	Fruits
41	Amalaki	Emblica officinalis Gaertn	Fruits
42	Bibhitakee	Terminalia bellirica Roxb.	Fruits
43	Mulaka	Raphanus sativas Linn.	Raddish
44	Erandakarkati	Carica papaya Linn.	Fruits
45	Chavya	Piper chava Hunter	Fruits
46	Guduchi	Tinospora cordifolia	Stem
47	Kulattha	Dolichos biflorus Linn	Seeds
48	Jiraka	Cuminum cyminum Linn	Fruits
49	Yavani	Trachyspermuanm ammi(L) Sprague	Fruits
50	Saileya	Parmelia perlata Ach.	Lichens
51	Kustha	Saussurea lappa C. B. Clarke.	Roots
52	Aguru	Aquilaria agallocha Roxb	Heartwood
53	Lavanga	Syzygium aromaticum (Linn)	Dried bud

54	Katuka	Picrorhiza kurroa Royle ex Benth	Roots
55	Shatapushpa	Anethum sowa Kurz	Fruits
56	Ativisha	Aconitum heterophyllum wall	Tubers
57	Kantakari	Solanum xanthocarpum	Root & other parts
58	Dhanyaka	Coriandrum sativum Linn	Fruits
59	Gapusha	Juniperus communis Linn	Fruits
60	Trivritta	Operculina turpethum	Roots
61	Ela-laghu	Elettaria cardamomum	Fruit – seeds
62	Nirgundi	Vitex negundo Linn.	Root, bark, Leaves
63	Mundi	Sphaeranthus indicus linn.	Herb
64	Snuhi	Euphorbia neriifolia Linn	Stem
65	Nimba	Azadirachta indica	Various parts
66	Aragvadha	Cassia fistula Linn	Pod, bark
67	Vacha	Acorus calamus Linn	Root
68	Bakuchi	Psoralea corylifolia Linn	Bark
69	Kanchanara	Bauhinia variegate Linn	Bark
70	Tvak-darusita	Cinnamomum zeylanicum	Bark
71	Patra	Cinnamomum tamala	Leaves

72	Jatiphala-Jatikosha	Myristica fragrans Houtt.	Fruit
73	Puga	Areca cateehu Linn	Nut
74	Danti	Baliospermum montanum	Seeds, Root
75	Bhringaraja	Eclipta alba Linn	Herb
76	Chirabilva	Holoptelea integrifolia	Bark
77	Apamarga	Achyranthes aspera Linn.	Seeds, Root
78	Bimbi	Coccinia indica	Fruits
79	Karanja	Pongamia pinnata (Linn.)	Bark, seeds
80	Mesasringi	Gynema sylvestre	Leaves
81	Saireyaka	Barleriaprionits Linn.	Herb
82	Sinsipa	Dalbergia sissoo Roxb.	Heartwood
83	Brihati	Solanum indicum Linn.	Root, various parts
84	KrisnajTraka	Carum carvi Linn.	Fruits
85	Kankola	Piper cubeba Linn	Seeds
86	Bola	Commiphora myrrh(Oleo-gum)	Resin
87	Damanaka	Artemisia sieversiana	Leaves, flowers, plant
88	Salaparni	Desmodium gangeticum	Root, whole plant
89	Chanaka	Cicer arietinum Linn.	Gram (seeds)
90	Kodrava	Paspalum scrobiculatum Linn.	Gram (seeds)

91	Indrayava	Holarrhena antidysenterica	Seeds
92	Madhavi	Hiptage benghalensis	Root-bark (Atimuktaka)
93	Misreya	Foeniculum vulgare Mill.	Fruits
94	Sarala	Pinus roxburghii Sargent	Wood
95	Karpura	Cinnamomum camphora	Extract
96	Lohavana-Loban	Styrax benzoin	Exudate-resin
97	Sthouneyaka	Taxus baccata Linn	Bark
98	Jatamansi	Nardostachys jatamansi DC	*Root*
99	Tinduka	Diospyros peregrina (Gaertn.)	Herb

Non-Herbal Drugs useful in Obesity

A. *Mineral/Metals etc.*

1.	Loha	:	Iron
2.	Maksika	:	Chalcopyrite
3.	Kasisa	:	Ferrous Sulphate
4.	Silajatu	:	Asphaltum
5.	Lavana	:	Salt
6.	Kantaloha	:	Kind of Iron
7.	Rasasindura	:	Sutabhasma
8.	Haratala	:	Orpiment
9.	Tamra	:	Copper
10.	Parada	:	Mercury
11.	Gandhaka	:	Sulphur

12.	Abhraka	:	Mica
13.	Tamra	:	Copper
14.	Mandura	:	Ferric Oxide
15.	Tahkana	:	Borax

B. *Animal Source*

1.	Madhu	:	Honey
2.	Kasturi	:	Musk
3.	Laksa	:	Lac
4.	Gomutra	:	Cow's urine
5.	Godugdha	:	Cow's milk
6.	Sankha	:	Conch shell

C. *Natural Source*

| 1. | Jala-ushna | : | water-hot |
| 2. | sukhoshna | : | lukewarm |

IMPORTANT FORMULATIONS

Sr.No.	Name of combination	Reference
1.	Chavyadi choorna	Bhavprakash 39/15
2.	Phalatrikadi choorna	Bhavprakash 39/16
3.	Vidangadi choorna	Bhavprakash 39/17
4.	Shilajatvadi Udvartana	Bhavaprakash 39/28
5.	Guduchyadi Kwath I	Bhavaprakash 39/23
6.	Brihatpanchamula Kwath	Bhavaprakash 39/18-19
7.	Karkashadi Kwath	Bhavaprakash 39/20
8.	Eranda Yoga	Bhavaprakash 39/21
9.	Gavedhukadi Prayog	Bhavaprakash 39/22

10.	Badari Peya	Bhaishajya Ratnavali, sthoulya 12
11.	Agnimantha Yoga	Bhaishajya Ratnavali, sthoulya 12
12.	Vyoshadya Saktuka	Bhaishajya Ratnavali, 6/8
13.	Amrutadya Guggulu	Bhaishajya Ratnavali, 13
14.	Lauha Rasayana	Bhaishajya Ratnavali 15/16
15.	Triphaladya Tailam	Bhaishajya Ratnavali 28/29
16.	Vadvagni Lauham	Bhaishajya Ratnavali, 45-46
17.	Tryushanadya Lauham	Bhaishajya Ratnavali 39-40
18.	Mahasugandhi Tailam	Bhaishajya Ratnavali 48-52
19.	Shirishadi Choorna	Bhaishajya Ratnavali 31
20.	Haritakyadi Pralep	Bhaishajya Ratnavali 33
21.	Haritala Yoga	Bhaishajya Ratnavali 34
22.	Dalajaladi Lepa	Bhav Prakash 36
23.	Alambusha Choorna	Bhav Prakash 36
24.	Vidangadya Lauham	Bhaishajya Ratnavali 41-42
25.	Loharishta	Bhavaprakasha, Bhaishajya Ratnavali, 56-60
26.	Lauhasava	Sharangadhar Samhita
27.	Kanchanar Guggulu	Bhaishajya Ratnavali 33-36
28.	Arogyavardhini Vati	Rasaratnasamuchchaya 28/106-108
29.	Vyoshadya Guggulu	Ashtanga Hridaya Chikitsa 21/49
30.	Mahalakshmivilas Rasa	Rasendrasarasangraha Kapharogchikitsa 17-19
31.	Taramandur Guda	Bhaishajya Ratnavali Shool Roga 108-109

32.	Pugakhanda	Bhaishajya Ratnavali Shool Roga 200-204
33.	Karpuradyarka	Arkaprakasha shataka 4, 18-22
34.	Avipattikara Choorna	Bhaishajya Ratnavali, amlapitta56, 25-26
35.	Mahayograj Guggulu	Bhaishajya Ratnavali, Vatvyadhi 24, 327-330
36.	Yograj Guggulu	Bhaishajya Ratnavali, 29, 156-159
37.	Brihatyograj Guggulu	Bhaishajya Ratnavali, Amavata, 29, 162-171
38.	Simhanada Guggulu	Bhaishajya Ratnavali, amavata, 29, 181-184
39.	Kubjavinoda Rasa	Bhaishajya Ratnavali, vatvyadhi.29, 131-132
40.	Amavateshvara Rasa	Bhaishajya Ratnavali, amavata, 29, 73-74
41.	Nyagrodhadi Kwatha	Sharangadhar Samhita
42.	Bilvadi Kwatha	Sharangadhar Samhita, Madhyam Khanda, 2,115-116
43.	Varunadi Kwath	Sushrut Samhita, Sootrasthana, 38
44.	Brihanmanjishthadi Kwath	Sharangadhar Samhita, Madhyam Khanda, 2, 137-141
45.	Tryushanadya choorna	Yog Ratnakar

46.	Madhutailika Basti	SG, UTTARAKHANDA, CHAPTER 8, 29-30
47.	Durgandhihara Yoga	SG, 117-118
48.	Durgandhaghna Yoga	SG, 118-119
49.	Patradi Pradeha	Charak Samhita, Sutrasthana, 3/29
50.	Vidangadi Churna	(CH.D.,B.R.,R.R.S.)
51.	Guduchyadi yoga	(Y.R., Basava.R.)
52.	Hingvadya choorna	(A.H.U)
53.	Guggulupanchapala choorna	(A.H.U)
54.	Vidangadya vataka	CH, D.
55.	Vidangadya Loha	Bhaishajya Ratnavali
56.	Vadavagni loha	Bhaishajya Ratnavali
57.	Tryvushanadya loha	Bhaishajya Ratnavali
58.	Vadavagni rasa	Yog Ratnakar
59.	Vadavagni rasa	Rasa Ratna Samuchchaya
60.	Agnikumara rasa	Rasa Ratna Samuchchaya
61.	Dashanga guggulu	Bhav Prakash
62.	Tryvushanadya guggulu	Bhav Prakash
63.	Vyoshadi guggulu	Ashtang Hridaya
64.	Agnimantha kwatha	Bhaishajya Ratnavali
65.	Patradi kashaya	Rasa Ratna Samuchchaya
66.	Vrandatriphaladyataila	Yog Ratnakar
67.	Haritakyadi Lepa	
68.	Samudraphena + Mocharasa	Yog Ratnakar
69.	Sthaulyantaka rasa	Basav Rajeeyam
70.	Trimurthi rasa	Basav Rajeeyam

71.	Shaileyadya Udvartan	Bhav Prakash
72.	Shireeshadi Udvartan	Bhaishajya Ratnavali
73.	Eranda patra kshara + Hingu	Bhav Prakash
74.	Loharasayana (CH.D.,B.R., V.S.)	Bhaishajya Ratnavali
75.	Haritala prayoga	Bhaishajya Ratnavali
76.	Eranda kshara prayoga	Bhaishajya Ratnavali
77.	Rasabhasma	Yog Ratnakar
78.	Trimurthi rasa	Yog Ratnakar
79.	Madhoodaka	Charak Samhita
80.	Madhumanda	Bhaishajya Ratnavali
81.	Madhwardraka prahoga	Ras Ratna Samuchchaya
82.	Chavyadi Yog	Bhaishajya Ratnavali
83.	Gandhaka yoga	Basav Rajeeyam
84.	Triphala Choorna	
85.	Mulaka Yoga	
86.	Manda Prayoga Manda / Saktu	
87.	Vasa swarasa + Shankha choorna	
88.	Haridra + Chincha swarasa	
89.	Guduchyadi Kwath II	
90.	Shaileyadi Udvartanam	
91.	Navaka Guggulu	
92.	Vasa- Bilva and Chinchadi Prayog	

93.	Lauha- Vanga- Vajra Bhasma	
94.	Triphala Kwath	
95.	Shirishadi pradeha	
96.	Chandraprabhavati	
97.	Mustadi Kwath	
98.	Guduchyadi Kwath II	
99.	Medodhwamsa rasa	
100.	Samshoshana rasa	
101.	Sthaulya gajakesari rasa	
102.	Sthaulyantaka rasa	
103.	Sthaulyaapakarshana rasa	
104.	Triphala kwatha	

Some Time Tested Drugs- Anubut Yog

- Herbs - कृष्णाजीरक, कंकोळ, दमनक, अग्निमंथ, भूर्ज, पारिभद्र, पटोल, पुष्करमूळ, वरूण, वासा, यव, शिग्रु, चित्रक, एरण्ड, गुग्गुळ, हरिद्रा, हरितकी, निंब मुस्ता, विडंग, रसांजन, देवदारू, काश्मरी, कारवेल्लक, मेथी, शुंठी, त्रिकटू, त्रिफला, पपई, गुडुची, चव्य, कुळीथ, जीरक, यवानी, कुष्ठ, अगरू, लवंग, कुटकी, शतपुष्पा, अतिविषा, कंटकारी, त्रिवृत्त, लघुएला, निर्गुण्डी स्नुही आरग्वध, वचा बाकुची कांचनार पूग, भृंगराज, अपामार्ग, करंज, शिंशपा, इंद्रयव, मिश्रेया, कर्पूर, जटामांसी, इंद्रवारूणी, श्यामाक. अतिमुक्त गवेधुक, माध्वी.
  Followed by honey later.
- मध + काललोह व यवक्षार यव + आमलकी
- बिल्वपंचमूल + मध   - अग्निमंथरस
- त्रिफला क्वाथ + मध   - शृतशीतजल + मध

- चव्य, जिरे, सुंठ, मिरी, पिंपली, हिंग, सौवर्चल, चित्रकमूळ चूर्ण समभाग + सातू + मध दीपन, लेखन.
- तालपत्रक्षार + शुद्ध हिंग + तंडुल मंड.
- फलत्रिकादि - त्रिफला, त्रिकटु - समभाग + तेल, सैंधव. ६ महिने सेवन कफमेद वातघ्न.
- गुडूची + मुस्ता/त्रिफला - तक्रारिष्ट/मध
- नवक गुग्गुल - त्रिकटु + त्रिफला + त्रिमद + गुग्गुळ.- मेद, कफ, आमवातघ्न.
- ½ tsp honey + ½ tsp basil leaves - paste in 1 glass of luke warm water to drink.
- 1 glass of water + soak 2 tablespoon of horse gram & keep it for a day.

- हरिद्रा - हरिद्रा उद्वर्तन.बब्बूल पत्र, हरितकीफल बदरीपत्र, बिल्वपत्र.
- भूर्जपत्र - कैयदेवनिघंटु.
- बीजक/असन - मध - उषःकाल - पान.
- तीलतैल - प्रातःकाल सेवन.
- त्रिफला इ मध/तक्र, निंब.
- सालसारादिगणचूर्ण + गोमूत्र - प्रातःकाल - पान.
- सूरणकंद + शुंठी + पाणी - लेपनार्थ

- **हरितकी + त्रिफला + तक्र + अरिष्ट**
- अग्निमंथ क्वाथ + शिलाजीत
- गुग्गुल +गोमूत्र + बृहत्पंचमूल क्वाथ/ अग्निमंथ क्वाथ
- चित्रकमूळ चूर्ण + मध.
- एरंडपत्रक्षार + हिंग – orally. only rice diet.
- रसांजन + बृहत्पंचमूल + गुग्गुल + शिलाजीत + अग्निमंथ.
- हरितकी + मध + सुरा.
- जम्बू क्वाथ.
- पटोलपत्रक्वाथ + चित्रकमूल_+ शतपुष्पा, हिंगु
- तांबूलपत्र +१० ग्रॅम मरिच - शीतजलासह. - अतिस्थूल व्यक्ती कृश होतो.

- एरंडपत्रक्षार + हिंग + तंदुलमंड
  Drink early morning on empty stomach.
  Soak leaves of jujube in water and keep solution overnight – drink on empty stomach in morning.
  Non herbal drugs.
- लोह, माक्षिक, कासीस, शिलाजीत, लवण, कांतलोह, रससिंदूर, हरताल, ताम्र, पारद, गंधक, अभ्रक, मंडुर, टंकण.
- मध, कस्तुरी, लाक्षा, गोमूत्र, गोदुग्ध, शंख.

CHAPTER 11

MANAGEMENT OF OBESITY - IN VIEW OF MODERN SCIENCE

Weight Loss Strategy

- A life-long eating plan for good health, which includes nutritionally adequate eating, reasonable expectations, regular physical activity, and permanent lifestyle changes, is best for achieving permanent weight loss.
- Weight loss of 0.5-2 pounds per week or 10% of body weight in six months is safe.

A Guide to Selecting Treatment

Treatment	BMI Category				
	25-26.9	27-29.9	30-34.9	35-39.9	≥ 40
Diet, exercise, & behavior therapy	With co-morbidities	With co-morbidities	+	+	+
Pharmacotherapy		With co-morbidities	+	+	+
Bariatric Surgery				With co-morbidities	+

It is Difficult to alter patient's expectations .
Unmet goals lead to

- Less satisfaction with treatment,
- Risk of drop-out
- Risk of regain
- Risk of depression

Should Unrealistic Expectations be Changed?

- The Theory

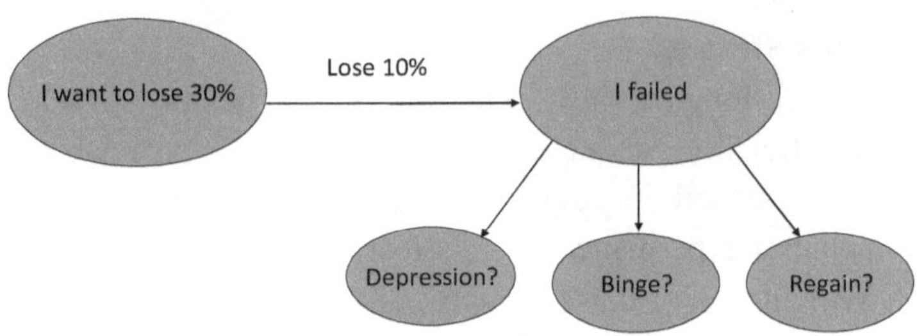

Setting Realistic Expectations

"The initial goal of weight loss therapy for overweight patient is a reduction in body weight of about 10%... Moderate weight loss of this magnitude can significantly decrease the severity of obesity-associated risk factors."

Set realistic goals.

- Weight-loss goals can be process goals, such as exercising regularly, or outcome goals, such as losing 20 pounds in four months.
- Make sure process goals are realistic, specific and measurable. For example, you'll walk for 30 minutes a day, five days a week.
- For outcome goals, aim to lose weight at a safe pace of 0.5 or 2 pounds a week. Losing weight more rapidly means losing water weight or muscle tissue, rather than fat.

Treatment Modalities

- Diet – (proper "Healthy" nutrition)
- Exercise
- Behavior therapy/modification/change
- Pharmacotherapy
- Surgery

Pharmacotherapy

Mechanism of drugs-

- Decrease lipid absorption
- Decrease energy intake
- Decrease pre-adipocyte differentiation and proliferation
- Decrease liogenesis and increase lipolysis.
- Modulation of carbohydrate metabolism
- Increase satiety
- Block dietary fat absorption
- Increase energy Expenditure
- Increase water elimination
- Enhance mood

Drugs - Weight-Loss Products

- Ephedrine-containing products inhibit serotonin and suppress the appetite. Supplements containing Ephedra have been banned by the FDA due to potential health risks.
- Herbal laxatives – These drugs do not prevent absorption.
- Sibutramine suppresses the appetite and is most effective when used with a reduced kcalorie diet and increased physical activity. There are many side effects.
- Orlistat blocks fat digestion and absorption. There are many side effects including anal leakage.

Anti obesity drugs act as anti-metabolites, capable of blocking pathway of oxidation of fatty acids. They alter either appetite, metabolism or absorption of calories.

Combinations- Melissa officinalis , Morus alba , Artemisia capillaries- for regulation of increased lipids.

Anti obesity drugs can act

- **Peripherally,**
- **Centrally or**
- **In combination.**

Peripherally acting-

1. Lipase inhibition-

Fat ------------------ intestine-------------------pancreatic lipase.

Drugs form covalent bond with active serine site of gastric and pancreatic lipases. Thus inhibiting the lipases from hydrolyzing ingested fat into absorbable free fatty acids and monoglycerides.

e.g.- Panax japonicus,   Platycordix radix   Salacia reticulata Tea- green, Oolong and Black, Nelumbo nucifera.

Theses herbs mainly include saponins, polyphenols, flavonoids and caffeine.

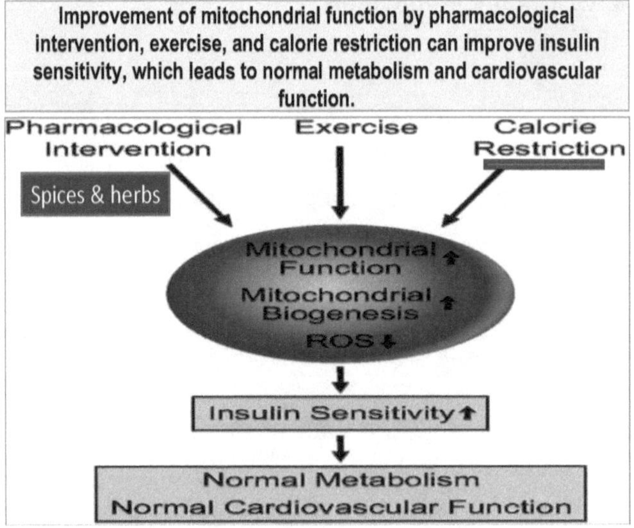

Adipogenesis down regulation-

Adipocytes primarily store triglycerides and release them in the form of free fatty acid with the change of energy demand in the body.

PUFAs (vital components of phospholipids of cell membranes) acts as signal transducer regulating adipocyte-specific gene expression involved in lipid metabolism and adipogenesis.

e.g. phytochemicals like quercetin kaempferol, catechin dietary flavonoids in vegetables, fruits, green tea and herbs are down regulate the adipogenesis related transcriptional factors PPAR and they inhibit adipocyte differentiation during early stage.

In addition to above, they show inhibitory activity against adipocyte differentiation, apoptotic effect on maturing pre-adipocytes; promoting fat mobilization.

2.   Thermogenesis-

BAT (brown adipose tissue) establishes non-shivering thermogenesis through dissipation of excess energy as heat. Important role in energy balance.

Searching for substances that upregulate UCP(mitochondrial uncoupling protein) gene expression may help in increasing energy expenditure.

e.g. ethanolic extract of solanum tubersome, caffeine, capsaicin.

4.   Lipid Metabolism-Stimulate triglyceride hydrolysis to diminish fat stores, by B3-ADRENERGIC RECEPTOR activation.

e.g. caffeine (oolong tea) nelumbo nucifera.

Centrally acting—

Effect on receptors in CNS to develop sense of satiety within body.

A] Neuropeptide signaling modulators-

Hormones are leptin, insulin, G1 peptide-ghrelin. Center for hunger is located in arcuate nucleus of hypothalamus.

1. Anorexigenic(hunger suppressants)
2. Orexigenic   (hunger stimulants) e.g. green tea

Neuropeptide Y (NPY)—increases hunger and weight.

e.g.- ginseng- decreases hunger and weight.

B] Monoamine neurotransmitters-

Alter hypothalamic neuropeptides at CNS. Alter key CNS appetite monoamine neurotransmitters levels to suppress appetite.

e.g. Green tea, Garcinia cambosia (natural hydroxy-citric acid- HCA), suppresses appetite.

Surgery

Surgery is an option for those who have tried weight loss programs and failed,have a BMI ≥ 35, and are having health problems due to their weight.

Gastric surgery has short-term and long-term problems and requires compliance with dietary instructions.

Liposuction is a popular procedure that is primarily cosmetic but poses risk.

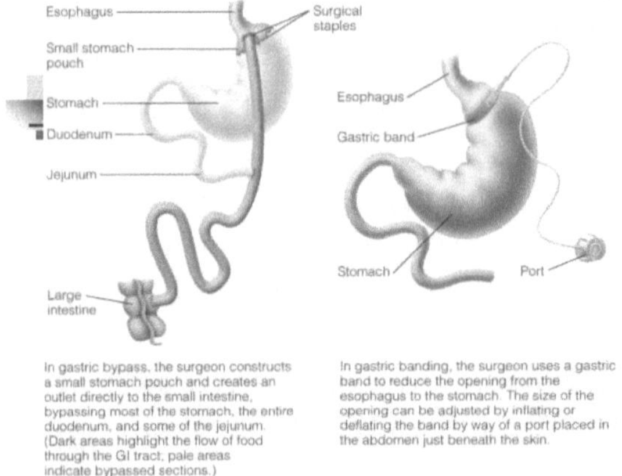

In gastric bypass, the surgeon constructs a small stomach pouch and creates an outlet directly to the small intestine, bypassing most of the stomach, the entire duodenum, and some of the jejunum. (Dark areas highlight the flow of food through the GI tract; pale areas indicate bypassed sections.)

In gastric banding, the surgeon uses a gastric band to reduce the opening from the esophagus to the stomach. The size of the opening can be adjusted by inflating or deflating the band by way of a port placed in the abdomen just beneath the skin.

Behaviour Therapy
Behavior modification

To lose weight and keep it off, one needs to make changes in lifestyle. But there's more to changing lifestyle than choosing different foods and putting more activity into day. It also involves changing approach to eating and activity, which means changing how we think, feel and act.

A behavior modification program can help make lifestyle changes.Behavior modification programs may include examining current habits to find out   what factors or situations may have contributed to excess weight. Exploring current eating and exercise habits gives a place to start when changing behaviors. Work out a strategy that will gradually change habits and attitudes. Consider how often and how long to exercise.

Determine a realistic eating plan that includes plenty of water, fruits and vegetables.

Write it down and choose a start date.

Behaviour Therapy

Behavior modification requires time and effort.

Awareness of behavior is the first key.

Changing behaviors one at a time works best.

Personal attitudes toward food and eating must be understood.

Support groups may be helpful for some people.

- Positive Affirmations Self esteem, Self confidence /efficacy,Good attitude, Positive outlook
- Strong Motivation
  Desire or want, Belief it is possible, Commitment to doing it Positive attitude, Persistence
- Supportive Environment
  Family and friends, Support group or organization, Professional help.
- Appropriate Behaviors
  Healthy eating, Exercise that produces goal, Changing problem behaviors

WEIGHT MAINTENANCE & PREVENTION OF WEIGHT GAIN

- Successful weight-loss maintenance programs use different criteria so they are difficult to compare.
- Vigorous exercise and careful eating plans are key.
- Frequent self-monitoring is recommended. Weekly weight, food diary, exercise journal, circumference measurements
- Eat regular meals and limit snacking.
- Drink water in place of high-kcalorie beverages.
- Select sensible portion sizes and limit daily energy intake to energy expended.
- Limit sedentary activities and be physically active.

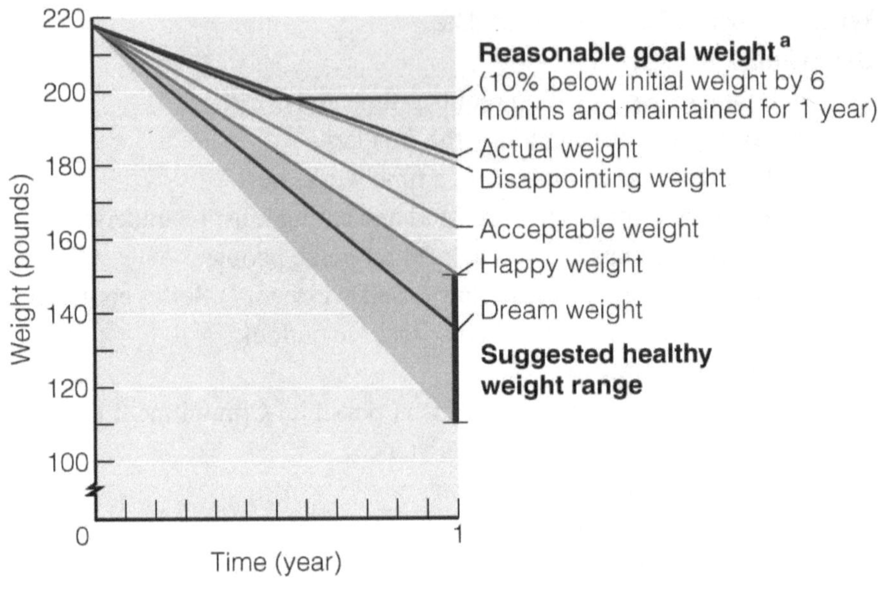
220
200
180
160
140
120
100
0
Weight (pounds)
Time (year)
0
1
Reasonable goal weight [a]
(10% below initial weight by 6
months and maintained for 1 year)
Actual weight
Disappointing weight
Acceptable weight
Happy weight
Dream weight
Suggested healthy
weight range

CHAPTER 12

STHAULYA – PATHYAPATHYA (DO'S & DON'TS FOR OBESITY)

SECRET OF HEALTH AND LONGEVITY

Eating correctly is life long commitment. Focus on essentials, eating right & eating on time. Otherwise body's starvation defenses will kick in lower metabolism and store fat.

FACTS ABOUT FAT

- More than 60% of the brain is composed of fat.
- 15% essential body fat is good and necessary.
- Functions of normal fat-
  heat insulation, keeps body moisturized
  absorption of shock (protects and nourishes bones)
  storage of energy(supply of energy in crucial states)
- Lean athletic body wt-More muscle mass& thickness, more bone density due to exercise, good diet leads to more weightbut lean, compact body
- More fat- more volume- more/less weighttruncal /general obesity.

GOOD DIET

- ✓ **Nutritionally adequate yet low in calories**
- ✓ **Fit into current lifestyle**
- ✓ **Foods that are liked**
- ✓ **Slow rate of weight loss**
- ✓ **Followed for life**

SOUND DIET

- Total kcal distribution –

Carbohydrates	–	50%
Proteins	–	20%

Fat   –   30%

- **Carbohydrates** – 45-65%
  emphases on complex forms as starch with fiber .
  Avoid simple sugar.
- **Proteins** – 10-35   lean food & small portions.
  Methionine (IAA) Indispensable amino acid
        To improve circulation of stored fats.
        To break it down into energy.
        Source – Quality protein like fish, eggs, whey, milk
         products.
        Whey protein, a powdered milk product has best
  biological value. Fish & eggs are better than chicken. Soy is great.
- **Fats**
  Consumption of MUFA : PUFA :SFA in the ratio of 1:1:1 is
   desirable.
  Total visible fat intake recommended /day = 10 gm (2tsp)
   equivalent to Mustard oil/Corn/olive oil (1tsp) +
   safflower/sunflower oil (1 tsp).
  **Saturated fat Ghee has short chain fatly acids these are easy
  to digest & promote good health.**
  Healthy fats – Nuts, cheese, ghee, paneer, fish.
  Oils of peanuts, olives, avocado, almond & rice bran .
  PUFA –Omega 6 – Sunflower, safflower (Kardai) soy bean oils.
  Omega 3 – flax seed, walnuts,beans, ghee, veg, nuts, oils in fish.
  Take equal amounts of omega 3 & 6.
  Trans fats – Bad fat, levels of low density lipo-protein or bad
   cholesterol.
  Processed foods, store – brought cakes, biscuits pizza, burger,
  fries.
       Fat = 10 gm/day
- **Water**
  Assist the body in metabolizing stored fat.
  Reduce sodium , fluid retention , fat deposits in the body.
  Helps to maintain proper muscles tone.

Rids the body of waste and toxins.

Relieves constipation.

Daily water intake of 2 to 3 ltrs. Is compulsory.

Requirement Changes according to water loss, Physical activity and special conditions.

Energy balance

- For adult male –
  Multiply body weight x10, add double body weight
  [for 150 1b – 1500 + (2x15 g) = 1800 cal/day
- For females
  150/b – 1500 + 150 = 1650 cal/day.
- Energy required for weight loss.
- Lifestyle   BMR + Lifestyle faster
- Sedentary   30% of BMR
- Moderate   50% of BMR
- Heavy   50% of BMR

Be Realistic about Energy Intake

> **300-500 kcalories/day reduction for BMI between 27 and 35**
>
> **500-1000 kcalories/day reduction for BMI ≥ 35**
>
> *Dietary Guidelines* should be followed.

<u>**HAVE DIET**</u> which is Bitter, pungent, astringent in taste, and dry, hot, sharp, scraping qualities

Whole grains- Barley, whole oats, bajri, nachni.

Vegetables-.

Pulses –Lentils, Mung dal, tu dar, masoor dal, horse gram chick peas

Fruits-

Honey

Spices-Fenugreek, turmeric, cumin, musturd, asefoetida, curry leaves, ginger,   black pepper, clove, cinnamon, Black jeera, Black   Til,Mustard   seeds,Coriander   seeds,Fennel seeds,Cinnamon,Cloves,Ginger, Hing & Turmeric, Black Pepper

USEFUL TIPS

- Maintain a regular daily routine.
- Take 2 teaspoon of honey and 2 tea spoon of lemon juice with 1 glass of warm water
- Exercise at morning at least 40 min/day -4days/week
- East light nourishing breakfast –cooked apple, toast cooked barley or oatmeal
- Cook daily with love and care
- Use spices and herbs that suitable for you while cooking
- Boil water with fresh ginger and drink frequently throughout the day
- Make Lunch as a main meal. Dinner should be as light as possible.
- For dinner, eat light one-dish meals, or vegetable or lentil soups.
- Do not sleep during day
- Keep the regular timings and correct quantity of meal. Eat mindfully.
- Eat only after digestion of previous meal. when you are hungry.
- Replace caffeinated and carbonated beverages with herb-spice teas.
- Avoid eating late at night
- Eat only after digestion of previous meal.
- Eat only when you are hungry. Find out correct quantity for you.
- Keep the regular timings of meal. Eat mindfully.
- Concentrate on your food, what you are eating. Don't divide your attention by reading, working or watching TV while you are eating.
- Take a walk after meal.
- Replace caffeinated and carbonated beverages with herb-spice teas.
- Fasting-One day fasting in a week is good
- Soups with no addition of fats or starch.
- Salad of raw tomato cucumber, cabbage capsicum, radish, lettuce green chilies, carrots, sprouted moong, Bengal grams.
- Avoid root veg like potato, beetroot.

- Avoid High calorie fruits like mangoes, bananas, dry fruits.
- Prefer Grilled/roasted/baked items than fried.
- cottage cheese than processed one.
- Avoid Alcoholic beverages.
- Limit cooking fat.
- Eat several mini-meals during the day, rather than three large meals. It helps one to avoid eating until they are "stuffed" and also reduces drops in the blood sugar levels.
- Fiber is excellent for weight loss and healthy too. which cleans out your system.
- Trim all fats from meats, remove skin from chicken.
- Before you put a snack or an extra helping in your mouth ask yourself. Am I Really hungry?
- If you get the urge to eat when not truly hungry Go for a walk Try to accomplish some small thing instead of going backwards on your diet.
- Regular exercise & smart use of carbohydrates lead to protein sparing. i.e. it is used for its intended purpose.
- Maintain a regular daily routine.
- Take 2 teaspoon of honey and 2 tea spoon of lemon juice with 1 glass of warm water
- Exercise at morning at least 40 min/day -4days/week
- East light nourishing breakfast –cooked apple, toast cooked barley or oatmeal
- Cook daily with love and care
- Use spices and herbs that suitable for you while cooking
- Boil water with fresh ginger and drink frequently throughout the day
- Make Lunch as a main meal. Dinner should be as light as possible.
- For dinner, eat light one-dish meals, or vegetable or lentil soups.
- Do not sleep during day
- Diet should be nutritionally adequate while avoiding excessive consumption.

- Smaller portions are recommended to feel satisfied, not stuffed.
- Eat foods of lower energy density, that are high in fiber, high in water and low in fat.
- Water is important to increase fullness and reduce hunger.
- Complex carbohydrates offer abundant vitamins, minerals and fiber with little fat.
- Choose fats sensibly and reduce the quantity of fat.
- Watch empty kcalories from sugar and alcohol.
- Plan meals throughout the day
- Eat a variety o Foods (at each meal)
- Center Meals around the carbohydrate foods
- Minimize the addition of FAT all the time and sugar at any one time
- Think about what you are going to eat instead of eating by habit or impulse!
- Eat more and earlier when more active
- Eat less and later when less active i.e. a little often vs. a lot at once
- The later you eat, the lighter you eat
- Variety of meal
  Provides more nutrition
  Each member of the family can choose what they want at that time
  Controls eating one food in excess
  Exposes a person to different foods
  Makes a better meal
- Minimize fats and sugar
  'Minimize' fat intake, don't eliminate it
   Sugar in <u>large amounts</u> is a problem
- Avoid food triggers. (Cues)
     Distract from the desire to eat with something positive
     Practice saying "No" to unhealthy foods and big portions.
     Eat when actually hungry — not when the clock says it's time to eat.

- Liaising with food industry to reduce energy of fat content & label

  Foods appropriately.
- Reasonable goal is to lose 10% of body weight
- Promoting healthy eating in schools
- Stomach can take amount of food that fits in our 2 palms at a time.
- Fruit sugar gets converted to triglyceride especially when eaten on a full stomach. Take as morning meal or after exercise.
- **WEIGHTLoss diets –**
- Reduction in daily energy intake of (600 kcal) from normal consumption.
- Goal - lose approx. 0.5kg/wk. compliance is improved by novelty of diet, so switch to a different dietary regime when weight loss slows on 1st diet.
- Vitamin. Supplementation if macronutrient balance is markedly disturbed.
- **VLCD– very low calorie diets. – Produce weight Loss of 1.5 – 2.5 kg/wk.**

Weight regains after stopping so Used for short term rapid weight loss.

- To minimize muscle degradation, Diet should ensure –

  Minimum-50 gm protein/D/for MALE,

  40 gm protein/D/for FEMALE

  Energy content should be minimum of

  - 400 kcal for female of ht < 1.73 m.

  -500 kcal for male and female of ht. >1.73 m

Pathya- Apathya-

There are series of food and edible items as well as activities of conducts which are favourable and considered wholesome for over-obese (ati-sthula purusHa) These may be put in two group :

A. Diet : Ahara

- Vataghna annapana

- Apatarpana-alpaharam (low quantity diet-non saturating food)
- Purana shaali
- Shleshmala medohara ahara

Uddalaka

Prashatika (Setaria italica)

Masoora

Priyangu (Aglaia roxburghiana)

Laja

Shyamaka (Echinochloa frumentosa)

Madhoodaka

Yavaka (Hordeum vulgere)

Arishta

Joornahva (Sorghum vulgere)

Sarshapa taila

Kodrava (Phaceolus mungo)

Takra

Kulatha (Dolichos biflorus)

Sura

Adhaki beeja (Cajanus cajan)

Chingata matsya

Patola (Trichosanthes cucumerina)

 Dagdha vartaku phala

Amalaka (Emblica officinalis)

Chakramudgaka

Puratana vainava (old rice)

Triphala (tried of three dug fruits viz. haritaki, bibhitaka and amalaki)

Guggulu

Ayash-lauha (iron)

Trikatu (tried of three purgent drugs viz. sunthi marica and pippali)

Pragbhojanasyapi vari pana

Anupan after food is-Madhoodaka—honey water, Arishta.

Ajeerna Manjiri

It is very nice concept in Ayurveda that resembles to concept of antidote in modern science. Herein, specific food material is advised for consumption after excess consumption of a particular food. It is believed and observed that this material nullifies side effects of over consumption of the food and protects body from that.

For e.g.-

- Coconut-rice
- Mango juice-milk
- Ghee-lemon juice
- Banana- ghee
- Wheat,maida, curds, alcohol, honey- cold water, cucumber
- Non-veg(mutton)- kanji, alcohol
- Sweets- warm water
- Jackfruit- banana
- Shrikhand- trikatu churna
- Jaggery- dry ginger+ khus powder
- Dry fruits (nuts)- clove(lavang)
- Fish- mango
- Buffalo milk and products- shankh bhasma
- Sugar- ginger

TIPS FOR WORKING WITH FAMILIES

1. Limit the intake of high calories snack foods
2. Avoid adding extra salt or salty foods
3. Limit the intake of pops, sodas, kool-aid, sweetened teas, Sunny Delight, fruit drinks/beverages, and other sugar based beverages
4. Model eating and exercising behaviors at home such as: drinking water, eating balance meals and eating fruits and vegetables
5. Support breastfeeding (parents, other family members, friends)
6. Increase the consumption of fruits and vegetables (fresh, frozen and canned {natural juices or light syrups})
7. Eat a variety of foods (meat, salads, fruits, vegetables, and water)

8. Take multi-vitamins daily
9. Encourage early prenatal visits and routine monthly visits, screening and Monitoring.

Alternative Low Cal Food

Item   Alternative
* Paratha (200 cal)   chapatti (80)
* Pulao/Biryani (170 cal/75gm)   Plain boiled rice (80 cal/75g)
* Fried Veg. (140/100gm0   Backed Veg (50/100gm)
* Fried/carried chicken/fish
* (250/135gm)   Grilled (160)
* Omelet (120 cal)   Poached/half boiled (60)
* Salad oil/mayonnaise   Lemon (0)
* (100 cal/Itbs/14gm0
* Sour meam (210/100)   Yoghurt (60)
* Regular sugar (20)   Caramelized sugar (5/13 p)
* Pudding 150   Fruit (40)
* Aerated soft drink (60-80)   Lime (0)
* Whole milk (170)   Skimmed (80/1 glass)
* Sharbat (80)   Buttermilk (40/1kg)

AHARA RUPI APATHYA

Madhura ,Sheeta Ahara
Shali
Godhooma
Ksheera Vikruti
Ikshu Vikruti
 Masha
Matsya
Mamsa
Bhojananantara Vari pana

DIET TO AVOID

- Avoid sweet, sour, salty and oily food as it aggravates Kapha and Meda
- Sweet foods include not only sugar but also rice, wheat, pasta, breads, and sweet milk products.
- Cakes, cookies, Pastries, Chocolates.
- Dairy products especially cheese cream, ice cream, yogurt.
- Meat especially red meat ,fried food ,grilled food
- Avoid packaged foods, processed food and restaurant fried foods - pizza, hot dog ,burger, doughnuts, French fries
- Avoid left over's
- **Avoid incompatible combinations of food**

  Milk with fish, meat, curd, sour fruits, bread containing yeast, cherries, yogurt

  Yogurt with milk, sour fruits, melons, hot drinks, meat, fish, mangos, cheese Eggs with milk, meat, yogurt, melons, cheese, fish, bananas Fruit with any other food
- **Avoid Tamasic food**

  Tamasic foods are those dull the mind and bring about inertia laziness disorientation depression.

  Excess intake of fats oils sugars, heavy and left over food are Tamasic in nature.

  Foods that have been processed, canned or frozen food , Beef, fish, eggs, cold buffalo milk are also Tamasic.
- **Crash diet** :- Once we are 'off' the diet, all our Wt is back & is only in terms of fat weight We lost muscle & bone density, & fat weight is higher than earlier.
- **Unsound diet**

  Promotes quick weight loss

  Limits food selection

Consequences of wrong dieting

- ➢ Decrease in rate of weight loss
- ➢ Loss of lean tissue with fat loss

- Decrease in metabolism, 10-40%
- Decrease in Protein turnover
- Preoccupation with food
- Increase in irritability, moodiness
- Tires easier, less physical activity
- Apathy, depression

Re-feeding after Weight Loss
- Increase in pre-dieting food intake,
- Preference for high fat foods
- Regain in weight, but greater increase in % BF
- Metabolism slow to return to normal, Regain Wt quicker with each diet
- Increase in abdominal fat deposits, Decrease in self-efficacy/esteem
- Less likely to return to pre-diet physical activity
- Decrease in self-efficacy/esteem

Vihara – Pathya – Do's

i) Chinta (worry)
ii) Shram (physical exertion)
iii) Jagarana (awakening)
iv) Vyavaya (coition)
v) Udvarttana
vi) Langhana (fasting/anti-saturation)
vii) Atapa (exposure to heat)
viii) Yanam (riding)
ix) Bhramana (walking)
x) Vireka- purgation
xi) cchardana - emesis

CHAPTER 13

STHAULYA CHIKITSA- VYAYAM (EXERCISE FOR OBESITY)

Vagbhata , in Ashtanga Sangraha, Sutrasthana chapter 3, verse no. 62-63 has defined Vyayama as----

Physical activity or bodily exertion which produces fatigue and tiredness in physique is defined as Vyayam (Physical exercise).it is considered an effective activity of human body for producing mainly-

1. Laghavam- Lightness Or Easiness
2. Karmasamarthya- Working Capacity
3. Deeptagni- Improvement In Gastric Power And Ultimately Digestion
4. Medakshaya- Decrease In Deposited Fat
5. Vibhakta Ghanagatratvam – Toning And Shaping Up Of Muscles
6. Ghanagatrata- Compactness Of Body Structures

Ardhashakti Vyayam-

Limit or extent of exercise is defined by Vriddha Vagbhata in Ashtanga Sangraha, Sutrasthana chapter 3, verse no. 64 as—

Person who is having good physical strength and consuming unctuous diet should perform physical exercise to the half of his physical capability during Visarga kala and less exercise in Aadana kala.

To get more benefits of Vyayam, Udvartana- powder massage should be done . it reduces and dissolves meda (Medasah Pravilayanam) and kapha, makes different organs stable especially firmness to limbs. Vayu, that is deranged is restored to its normal condition. Utsadan and udgharshana dilates openings of sira i.e. channels and increase the temperature of the skin.

Vyayama is considered as one of the types of Anagni sweda. Vyayam is also considered as one of ten types of Langhan chikitsa.

Exercise

'Stop Dieting and Start Moving'

Exercise does not significantly increase initial weight loss over and above that obtained with diet only. However, **the diet plus exercise plan achieves more weight loss than the diet alone condition."**

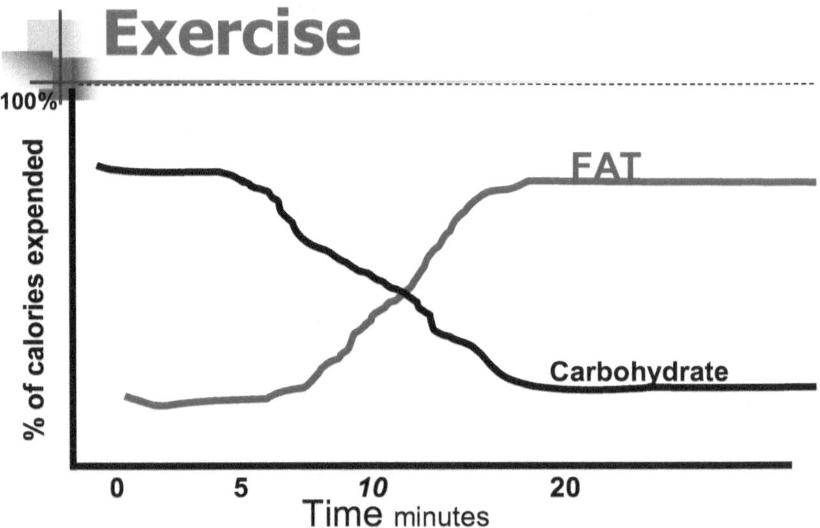

Physical Activity

- An individual's body weight as well as intensity and duration of activity influence energy expenditure.
- Physical activity increases the amount of discretionary k calories that can be consumed.
- Metabolic rates can rise with daily vigorous activity.
- Activity can decrease body fat and increase lean body mass.
- Exercise may help to curb appetite.
- Activity can reduce stress and improve self-esteem.

Choosing Activities

- Choose activities that you enjoy and are willing to do regularly.
- Low to moderate intensity for long duration is recommended.
- Daily routines can incorporate energy activities.
- Spot Reducing
- Regular aerobic exercise and weight loss will help trouble spots.
- Strength training can improve muscle tone.
- Stretching can help flexibility.

Physical And Psychological Activity .

- Metabolic rates can rise with daily vigorous activity.
- Activity can decrease body fat and increase lean body mass.
- Activity can reduce stress and improve self-esteem.
  - Strength training can improve muscle tone.
  - Stretching can help flexibility.

Points to remember about Exercise-

- 20-30 minutes of moderate exercise 5 to 7 days a week, preferably daily. Types of exercise include Walking stationary bicycling, walking or jogging on a treadmill, stair climbing machines, jogging, and Swimming.
- Exercise can be broken up into smaller 10-minute sessions.
- Start slowly and progress gradually.
- With use, muscles consume energy derived from both fat and glycogen. Due to the large size of leg muscles, walking, running, and cycling are the most effective means of exercise to reduce body fat. Exercise affects macronutrient balance. Signs that encourage the use of stairs as well as community campaigns have been shown to be effective in increasing exercise in a population.
- Maintenance of high physical activity levels by walking, cycling, swimming. (Maximize physical activity with reference to modest extra activity required to increase PAL (Physical activity level) ratios.

- PAL – <u>Total energy expenditure</u>
  BMR

Types of Exercise-
1. a]Static b] Kinetic
2. a] Aerobic b] Anaerobic

Main exercises in our routine life are- Walking, Swimming, running, or rowing aerobic exercises, Stationary Cycling/Bicycling. **Due to the large size of leg muscles, walking, running, and cycling are most effective means of exercise to reduce body fat.**

Exercises as per Prakruti (Constitution) and Dosha Vitiation-
- Kapha - Vigorous Exercises and activities like Running, Dancing, Hiking, Swimming, Triathlons, Brisk walking,
- Pitta - Challenging and vigorous hikes and treks in nature, competitive sports, swimming, Stationary Cycling/Bicycling
- Vata - Movement with gentle pace- Yoga, light amount of Dance aerobics and resistance training(weights),Stretching.

YOGA

It includes-Asana, Pranayam, Mudra, Bandha, Dhyan
1. **Asana – Specific Postures.**

Asanas are specifically mentioned for offering Sthairya, Aarogya, Angalaghavam and Dridhata. Main asanas useful for treating obesity are- Utthanpadasana , Dvichakrikasan, Padvruttasan, Naukasana, Viparitakarni mudra, Halasana, Dhanurasana, Shalabhasana, Pawan muktasana, Makarasan, Tiryak Bhujangasan, Yashtikasan, Katichakrasan, Trikonasan, Pashchimottanasana, Yogmudra, Matsyasana, Ushtrasana, Ardhamatsyendrasana, Vakrasana, Supta vajrasana, Gomukhasan, Parvatasan, Janushirasan, Marjarasan, Bhadrasan, Salambakokilasan,
Tadasan etc.

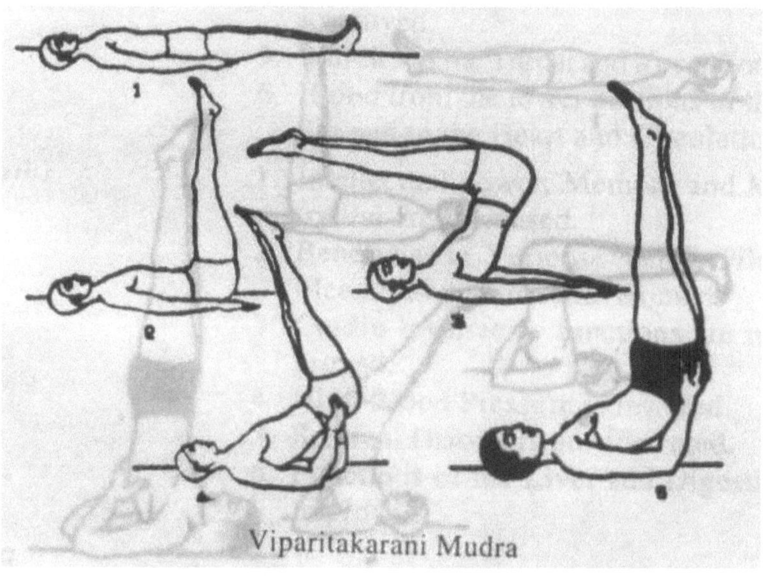

Viparitakarani Mudra

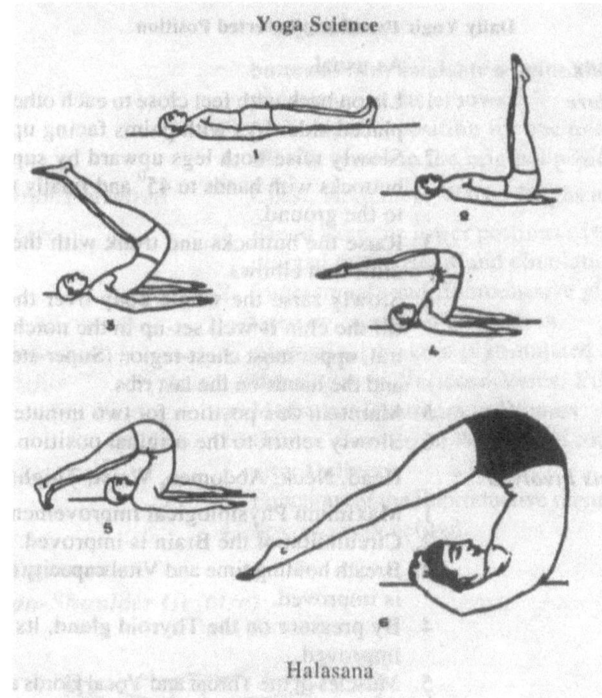

Halasana

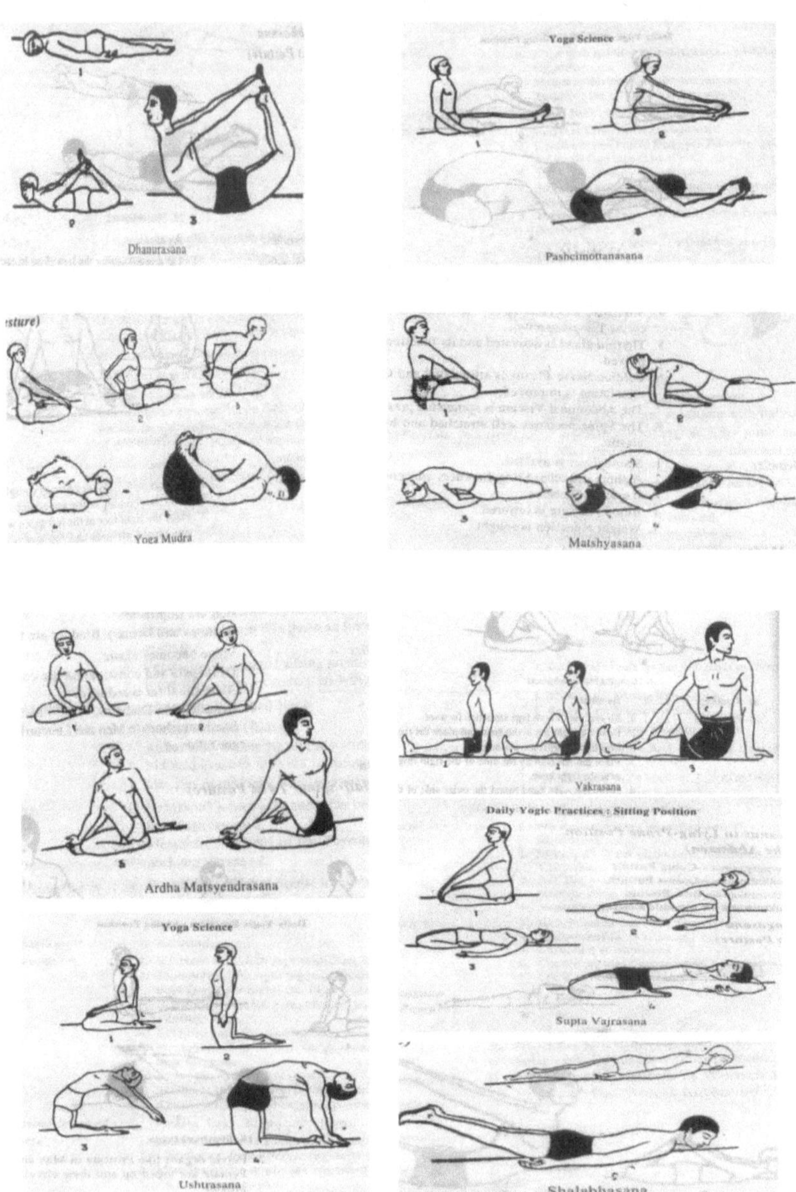

1. Viparita karani, Sarvangasana - Regulates functioning of endocrines like Thyroid and Pituitary.
2. Dhanurasana, Matsyendrasana - decreases abdominal deposition of fat through stretch receptor stimulation, improve muscle tone and muscle power to strengthen musculoskeletal system
3. Tadasana- maintains mind- body balance to increase self consciousness, self awareness and self realization strengthens abdominal muscles and shapes up abdomen.
4. Paschimottanasana - eliminates possibility of sciatica, decreases tension of thigh and calf muscles and makes them flexible.
5. Vrikshasanahelps to remove all the strain.

2. Pranayam and Dhyan –
Breathing Exercises and Meditation –

Ultimate outputs of pranayama and especially AUM chanting are Kayasya krishata, Kanti, Agni pradeepan, Laghavam, Nirlepan). They do Correction of metabolism through regulation of Vata dosha. Bhasrika, kapalbhati and suryabhedan pranayam are useful.

a. bhasrika- good to remove sluggishness of body. Corrects depletion of prana. Normalizes vitiated kapha. Good for digestive disorders.
b. Kapalbhati- decreases fat of abdominal area. Decreases adipose tissue of abdomen and greater omentum. Useful in elimination of excessive kapha

3. Mudra – Specific postures of specific body parts. Different mudras offers Sthairya to physique and psyche. Sinha mudra is specially useful for treating obesity.

4. Bandha – it is Holding of body, breath and mind in specific postures.

5. **Surya Namaskar** – Sun Salutations

It is an active and dynamic series that exerts its major influence on Pingala Nadi and all Chakras. It generates heat effect rather thermal axis of body deviates towards heat. So, its physiological function is seen as increased BMR. All major groups of muscles get exercised by 12 postures of Suryanamaskar.

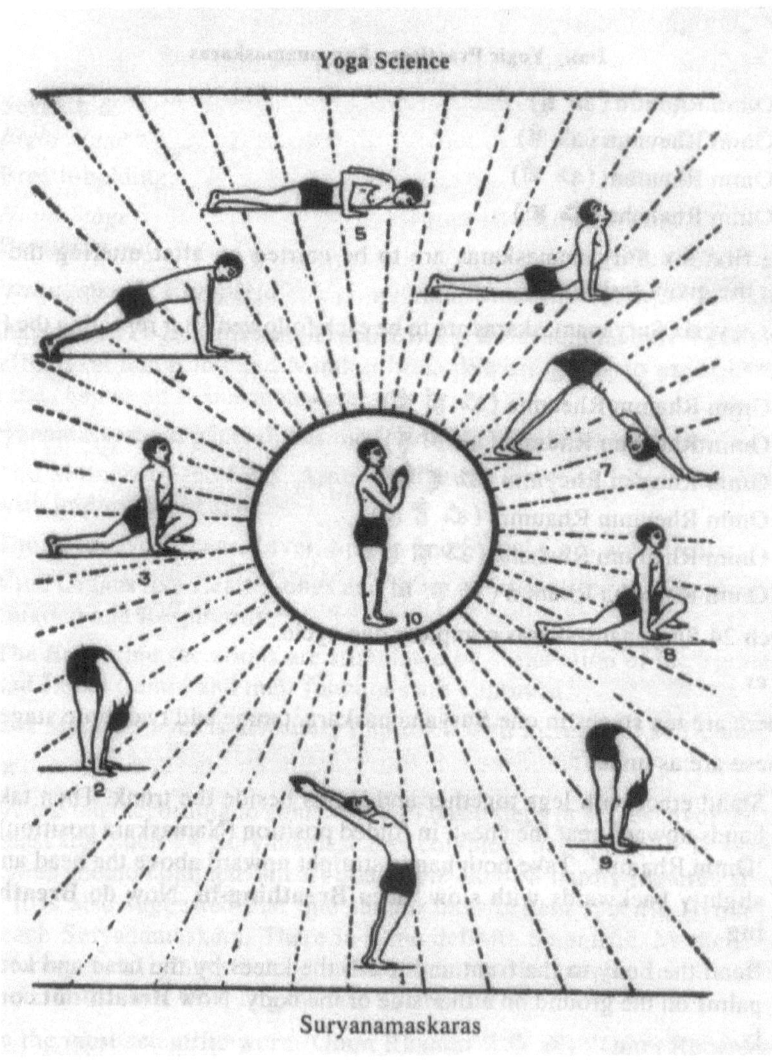

Suryanamaskaras

REFERENCES

➢ Charaka Samhita Sutra Sthana 21st Ch.(Ashta ninditiya Adhyaya)

➢ Sushruta Samhita Sutra Sthana 15th Ch.
(Dosha Dhatu Mala vrudhi Vijnaneeya Upakrama)

➢ Ashtanga Hrudaya Sutra Sthana 14th Ch.
(Dwividhopakramaneeya adhyaya)

➢ Bhela Samhita Sutra Sthana 11th Ch.

➢ Vangasena Samhita 16th Ch.(Medoroga)

➢ Madhava Nidana 34th Ch.(Medoroga)

➢ Bhava Prakasha 34th Ch.

➢ Yoga ratnakara Medorogaadhyaya

➢ Chakradatta 36th Ch.

➢ Gadanigraha 13th Ch.

➢ Bhaishajya Ratnavali 39th Ch.

➢ Rasa Ratna Samuchaya 18th Ch.

➢ Dr.V.B.Athavale, Obesity in Ayurved

➢ Dr. Anaya Pathrikar, Asti Sthoolasya Bheshajam
– Obesity – concept to cure

➢ Howie, L.D., ADA, 2003;103:1653-1657

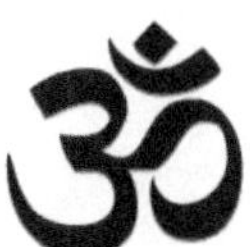

सर्वे भवन्तु सुखिनः सर्वे सन्तु निरामयाः।
सर्वे भद्राणि पश्यन्तु मा कश्चिद्दुःखभाग् भवेत्।।

May all be happy; May all be free from infirmities;
May all see good; May none partake suffering.